Surgical Mayo
Setups

Surgical Mayo Setups

Second Edition

Tammy Allhoff, AAS, CST/CSFA
Pearl River Community College
Surgical Technology
Program Director and Clinical Coordinator

Debbie Hinton, BS, CST
Pearl River Community College
Surgical Technology
Former Program Director

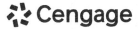

Australia • Brazil • Canada • Mexico • Singapore • United Kingdom • United States

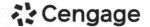

Surgical Mayo Setups,
Second Edition
Tammy Allhoff and Debbie Hinton

Vice President, Editorial:
Dave Garza

Director of Learning
Solutions: Matthew Kane

Senior Acquisitions Editor:
Tari Broderick

Managing Editor:
Marah Bellegarde

Senior Product Manager:
Juliet Steiner

Editorial Assistant:
Nicole Manikas

Vice President, Marketing:
Jennifer Baker

Marketing Director:
Wendy Mapstone

Senior Marketing Manager:
Michele McTighe

Marketing Coordinator:
Scott A. Chrysler

Production Director:
Wendy Troeger

Production Manager:
Andrew Crouth

Content Project
Management:
PreMediaGlobal

Senior Art Director:
Jack Pendleton

For product information and technology assistance, contact us at
**Cengage Customer & Sales Support, 1-800-354-9706
or support.cengage.com.**

For permission to use material from this text or product,
submit all requests online at **www.copyright.com.**

Library of Congress Control Number: 2011939225

ISBN-13: 978-1-111-13818-9
ISBN-10: 1-111-13818-4

Cengage
200 Pier 4 Boulevard
Boston, MA 02210
USA

Cengage is a leading provider of customized learning solutions with employees residing in nearly 40 different countries and sales in more than 125 countries around the world. Find your local representative at: **www.cengage.com.**

To learn more about Cengage platforms and services, register or access your online learning solution, or purchase materials for your course, visit **www.cengage.com.**

Printed in the United States of America
Print Number: 13   Print Year: 2022

Dedication

I would like to dedicate this book in honor of Debbie Hinton. She was a great leader, co-worker and teacher. But most of all, she was a very special friend.

As a leader, Debbie led by example. As an instructor, she taught with a style unique to her calm demeanor and with compassion for our students. As a co-worker, she was my rock and my example.

To all of our former students, you are truly blessed to have been taught by Debbie, because she was one of the best instructor's ever. To future students, I will try always to do my best to help you succeed and show compassion because I was trained by one of the best mentors ever in Debbie.

Debbie and I accomplished many things together. We produced many great surgical technologists, authored a series of surgical instrument modules and co-wrote the first edition of this book. But I feel that our greatest professional accomplishment was displayed in the teamwork that we brought to our classroom for over 16 years. I am so grateful and blessed to have been part of that team with Debbie and I am honored and humbled to carry on her legacy.

I will never forget her laughter, support, compassion, calmness and her love of surgical technology.

To her husband, Ben, and her son, Stuart, thank you so very much for sharing Debbie with me and our students for so many years. Her love of surgery and teaching was ever present and only surpassed by her love for you two guys.

For my husband, Ben, and my son, Stuart, for all their love and support. And to my mother, Betty Stuart, who gave me a passion for surgical technology.

Debbie

To my sons, Nick and Brad, who are my greatest accomplishment. Thank you for making my role as a parent so rewarding and fun. Always believe that you can achieve anything.

Tammy

And a special thanks to our students and colleagues who help make this profession fun, challenging, and, most of all, rewarding.

Debbie and Tammy

Table of Contents

Preface

Surgical Mayo Setups, 2nd Edition, is designed to be a basic guideline to Mayo tray setups for surgical team members who are preparing for procedures. The Mayo tray setup contains the surgical instrumentation commonly used during the surgical procedures. This book gives the operating room (OR) personnel who will be working in scrub roles, such as surgical technologist and surgical nurses, an overview of the surgical instruments and equipment needed to perform different procedures.

This book can be used as a baseline reference for experienced personnel. It will aid students who are training to perform in these roles. It can also be used by new personnel as a basic guideline for setups on specialty procedures they may not have experience with. Mayo setups and instrumentation vary according to facility, instrument set, and specialty procedure. Instruments may be given "slang" names at different facilities. This book contains proper names of instruments so it can be utilized nationwide. It can be of benefit to new employees, employees who have to cross-train in different specialties, and traveling scrub personnel. Cross-training is necessary because of the increase in types of surgical procedures being performed. Some facilities utilize traveling scrub personnel for various reasons, so this book can be a guide for them regarding unfamiliar procedures. Personnel that specialize in specific areas may also use this book as a reference when they are assigned to procedures outside of their specialty.

The book is divided into chapters by specialty procedure. The second edition begins with a new first chapter devoted to photographs of different variations of Mayo setups. It also includes photographs of setups that do not utilize a Mayo tray, but where the scrub person will instead work from the back table. The basic setup will be on the back table and this will be "pulled" up to the sterile field so that the most commonly used instruments are accessible.

Conceptual Approach

Having worked in the field of surgery, the authors felt a need for this type of book for many reasons. Specialized teams are being utilized more often now in the operating room. However, because of scrub personnel's specialization, they often need guidelines on setups that they may encounter when they are assigned out of their specialty field.

Also, because traveling scrub personnel may be assigned to a variety of specialty procedures at new facilities, the need exists for a reference to basic setups in all of the specialties. The scrub person can use this book to have a basic setup to follow in multiple specialties. Every surgeon has certain instruments he or she uses for specific reasons, and the scrub person can adjust the basic setup to include this specific instrumentation.

Students have a basic knowledge of setups when they begin their clinical rotations. This book can be used to instruct students on setups needed for a multitude of specific procedures in which they have no experience. If students begin their day or procedure with an efficient setup and level of confidence in their setup, it tends to make the procedure go more smoothly, and thus benefits everyone involved.

Organization

This book is divided into 13 chapters. The first chapter is a new feature containing photographs of different methods of setting up basic procedures. Variations include having the "roll towel" with instrumentation on one side or on the end of the Mayo tray. Photographs also include the variation of having a second Mayo setup that includes retractors needed during a procedure in which a cavity is opened. This allows the scrub person to be more organized with the primary Mayo setup. Another variation is the utilization of a setup on the back table, due to limited space surrounding the sterile field or limitations due to the position of the patient. Some specialty procedures or patient positions will also allow the scrub person to utilize a primary setup with a Mayo tray or a back table, depending on that person's preference and the layout of the operating room.

The other 12 chapters each cover a surgical specialty, and specify basic Mayo setups for that specialty. Surgical specialties included are: general; obstetric/gynecologic; genitourinary; thoracic; cardiovascular; peripheral vascular; orthopedic; neurological; plastic and reconstructive; ear, nose, and throat; ophthalmic; and oral/maxillofacial. This edition includes more than 150 basic Mayo setups for surgical specialties, as well as references to many other procedures. The AST level and specialty are provided for each procedure, so students will now also be able to distinguish the level and specialty according to AST guidelines.

Features

A handy, pocket-sized reference, *Surgical Mayo Setups, 2nd Edition,* has several key features designed to help all operating room personnel who work in a scrub role find the information they need as quickly and easily as possible.

- Contains more than 150 surgical Mayo setups
- Reference for many other procedures
- Tabbed for quick reference
- Contains proper names for instruments for universal application
- "Personal Notes" sections in each chapter allow space for note taking.
- Clear illustrations with labels help users visualize the setups for more complicated procedures.

New to This Edition

As mentioned, this edition includes a new introductory chapter providing crisp photographs of different basic Mayo setups. Included in this chapter are variations on a basic Mayo setup that users can adapt or adjust according to their specific needs. Some procedures that have a cavity open, such as the abdominal cavity, require more instrumentation.

Therefore, to organize efficiently, the scrub person can utilize a second Mayo setup to accommodate the larger retractors and specialty items needed.

AST has specific requirements for students during their clinical experience regarding case levels and specialties. In the new edition, each procedure is labeled according to its specialty and case level. This addition benefits student users in completing their required number of procedures and required levels during their clinical experience. It may also help new employees during their orientation process.

Twenty procedures have been added and cross-referenced to other procedures that can be performed with the same setup with a few variations. This will help the user during new assignments or cross-training in other specialties.

About the Authors

Debbie Hinton was a Certified Surgical Technologist with a BS in education. Mrs. Hinton was the Program Director and instructor for the Surgical Technology Program at Pearl River Community College in Hattiesburg, Mississippi. During her work experience in the field, she specialized in orthopedic and neurological procedures. She had more than 18 years experience in the field of education.

Tammy Allhoff is a Certified Surgical Technologist and Certified Surgical First Assistant. She has her Associate's Degree in Applied Science and is the Program Director and Clinical Coordinator with the Surgical Technology Program at Pearl River Community College. During her work experience in the field, she worked on the first open-heart team in Hattiesburg; worked as a CST, CSFA for a group of general, thoracic, and vascular surgeons; and then specialized in peripheral vascular surgery and worked as a Certified First Assistant. Mrs. Allhoff has more than 16 years in the field of education.

Both have also co-authored a series of computer programs on instrument trays for different surgical specialties, *Surgical Instruments* (Watson Enterprises).

Mrs. Allhoff is an active member in the Association of Surgical Technologists. During her life, Mrs. Hinton was an active member as well in the association.

Acknowledgments

We appreciate the help and sharing of knowledge from our colleagues in the field. This profession is both demanding and stressful and we would like to acknowledge all those who remain dedicated. We would also like to thank the surgeons with whom we have worked and who work with students. It takes special people to remember what it was like to be new to or unfamiliar with certain specialties. We would also like to thank the following reviewers:

L. Gene Burke, CST, AAS
Director of Surgical Technology
Augusta Technical College
Augusta, GA

Carolyn Ragsdale, CST, BS
Surgical Technology Program Director and Faculty
Parkland College
Champaign, IL

John D. Ratliff, CST, FAST, BS
Program Chair, Surgical Technology Program
York Technical College
Rock Hill, SC

Joseph Milam, CST, CRCST, AA, AS,
Program Director, Surgical Technology Program
Virginia College
Jacksonville, FL

Introduction

This book is designed to be a basic guide to follow when setting up Mayo trays. The exact instrumentation needed will depend on the facility, the surgeon's preference, and the type of procedure. Surgical instruments come in various sizes and lengths. The particular ones to be used on a procedure will depend on the size of the patient and the procedure(s) to be performed. For example, on an exploratory laparotomy, you may not always need the long Metzenbaum scissors and long forceps.

Also, many supplies are not placed on the primary Mayo tray, but instead are left on the back table where they are easily accessible during the procedures. This is necessary because of the limited room on the Mayo tray and the variations in a particular surgeon's preference as to retractors and other instruments. An example of this is needle holders. Various types are available, but they are all traditionally left on the back table so that they may be conveniently placed beside sutures, ready for use.

Most general surgery procedures, and many other types of specialty procedures, also require the use of various suture materials and ties. These are usually placed on the Mayo tray under a towel for easy access during the procedure. The ties to be used will depend on the specific procedure and the surgeon's preference.

Because of the nature of some procedures, you will find notes on the setup pages that some people choose to use a second Mayo tray for specialty clamps and retractors. This is also because of the limited space on a Mayo tray. You can find a photographic example of this in Chapter 1. Some procedure setups may also require the use of an extra-large table, called a *Mayfield*, because it can accommodate more instrumentation and supplies.

Variations on the basic Mayo setup can be made as desired, and different methods can be utilized for placement of instrumentation on the Mayo tray. Some scrub personnel choose to place their instrumentation on the end rather than one side of the tray. Various photographs demonstrating some of these methods appear in Chapter 1.

Surgical sponges are also sometimes placed on the Mayo tray so that the scrub person can promptly exchange soiled ones for clean ones during the procedure. Take the precautions necessary to keep an accurate count of all supplies before and during the procedure.

You can use the "Personal Notes" section at the end of each specialty chapter for making notes and recording tips on variations according to your facility or personal likes and dislikes. We recommend that you find a specific way that works for you and that can easily be taken over by relief personnel. Once you establish your way of setting up, it will expedite preparation for other procedures and give you confidence in your routine.

This book will provide a new employee or inexperienced scrub person with a basic idea of what specific instruments or supplies to place on a Mayo tray for procedures. It can also be used for personnel who are filling in or rotating through specialties other than their usual assigned areas. Because of specialty cross-training, some scrub personnel may be familiar with other setups. These setups can be used as a guide to prepare Mayo setup trays. There may be adjustments and variations for specific facilities' instrumentation trays and each surgeon's specialty instruments.

This book is not meant to replace the knowledge and expertise of the people who work in these specialties. It is professional and courteous to share knowledge and expertise with others so that we can reach the ultimate goals of giving high-quality patient care, expediting surgical procedures, and meeting the high demands and anticipation of the surgeon's needs. The information in this book should give the scrub person some degree of confidence for scrubbing on a variety of surgical specialties and procedures.

Specific protocol should be followed on all surgical procedures to ensure that the correct procedure, correct side, and correct patient policies are followed. Most facilities utilize the "Time out" standard, so this protocol should be adhered to at all times. Doing so protects all surgical patients and operating-room staff, surgeons, and facilities from performing procedures on the wrong patient or side.

Chapter 1

Setup Methods

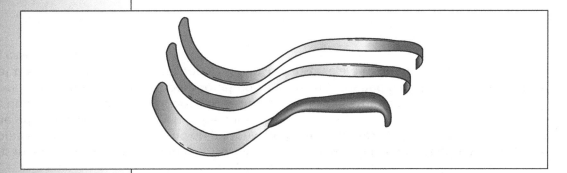

Introduction

There are many variations in regard to setting up a Mayo. The variations used will depend on specialty, procedure, facility, and OR layout. Some variations will also depend on personal preference. Setups are further dependent upon the site of surgery and the side on which the surgery is to be done.

Most sterile setups are done farthest from the OR door, to reduce traffic in and around the sterile setup. The following photos show different ways that you may choose to set up your instruments and back table. The photos are not meant to suggest that these are the only ways for you to set up, but instead are to be used as a guide for variations to make your setup easier to work from.

Examples of Basic Mayo Setups

Figure 1-1 shows the basic Mayo setup for exploratory laparotomy. Instrumentation can be adjusted according to the procedure being performed.

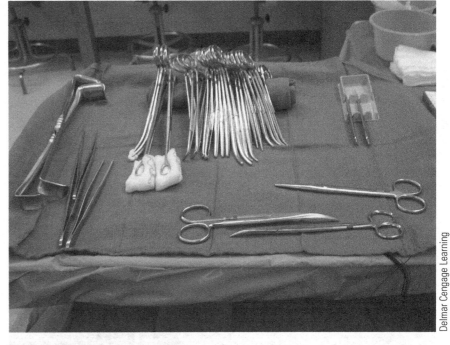

Delmar Cengage Learning

Figure 1-1: Basic Mayo setup for exploratory laparotomy

Figure 1-2 presents the basic Mayo setup including back table and ring basin. Scrubbed personnel would stand within the sterile area and have access to all instrumentation and supplies on the back table. The ring basin could be used for instrumentation that is no longer usable or needed, for sterile trash, or when breaking down the setup. It could also be used for large specimens. During the initial setup, the draping supplies (in order of usage) may be stacked here with the surgeon's gown and gloves on top.

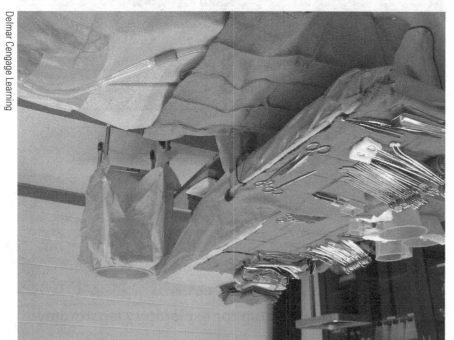

Delmar Cengage Learning

Figure 1-2: Basic Mayo setup including back table and ring basin

Figure 1-3 shows the basic back table setup with "working end" to be pulled up to a sterile field that includes the Mayo setup and the draped patient.

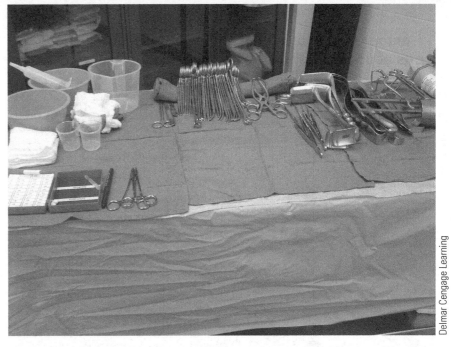

Delmar Cengage Learning

Figure 1-3: Basic back table setup with "working end"

Figure 1-4 shows a basic Mayo setup with the loaded sponge sticks and dissectors placed so that there will be room for other instrumentation to be added to the Mayo. The loaded scalpels are placed in a protective device for safety. The scrubbed personnel would stand near the end where the scalpels are located.

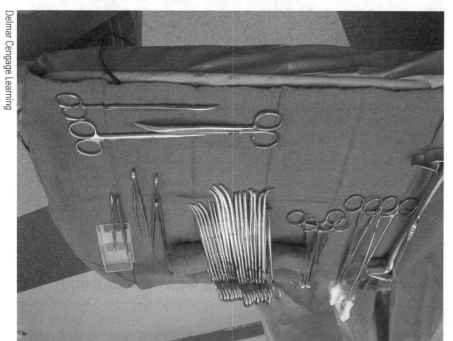

Delmar Cengage Learning

Figure 1-4: Basic Mayo setup with the loaded sponge sticks and dissectors, allowing room for additional instrumentation

Figure 1-5 presents a variation of a basic Mayo setup.

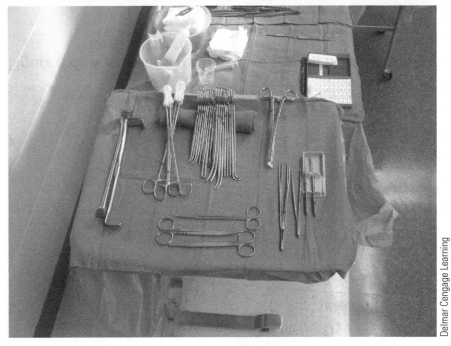

Figure 1-5: Variation of a basic Mayo setup

Delmar Cengage Learning

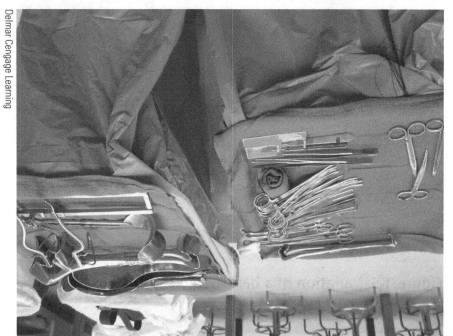

Delmar Cengage Learning

Figure 1-6: Basic Mayo setup with a second Mayo setup for large retractors

Figure 1-6 shows a basic Mayo setup with a second Mayo setup for large retractors. This variation can be used when there is a need for additional large retractors, as for procedures requiring multiple sizes and types of retractors.

Figure 1-7 shows a basic Mayo setup with roll towel for instrumentation placed at the end. This layout variation is sometimes used for different specialties, and instrumentation will also vary according to the specialty instrumentation required. The scrubbed personnel would stand at the opposite end of the roll towel and face the instrumentation on the roll towel.

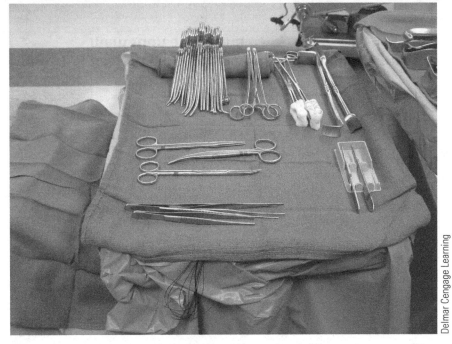

Delmar Cengage Learning

Figure 1-7: Basic Mayo setup with roll towel for instrumentation

Figure 1-8 presents the basic Mayo setup with the roll towel of instrumentation on the end of the Mayo stand. The second Mayo stand holds large retractors and is also sometimes used for specialty items, depending on the procedure. This basic setup includes large handheld retractors.

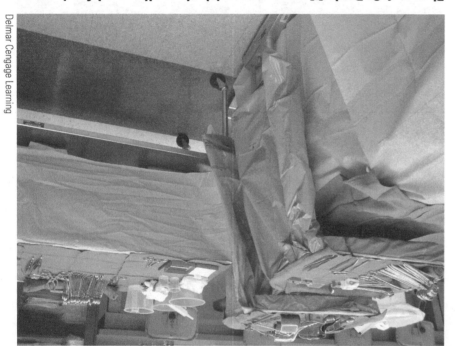

Delmar Cengage Learning

Figure 1-8: Basic Mayo setup with the roll towel for instrumentation at the end

Figure 1-9 shows a basic back table with the retractors left in the pan for organization and counting.

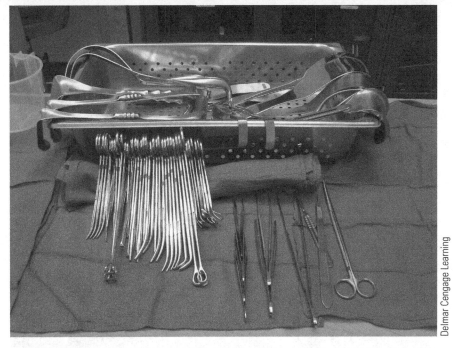

Delmar Cengage Learning

Figure 1-9: Basic back table with retractors left in the pan for organization and counting

Figure 1-10 demonstrates a basic Mayo setup for arm/wrist procedures. A back table can be used for the setup and pulled up to the sterile field, or a Mayo stand can be used with the back table pulled up along the back of the Mayo setup.

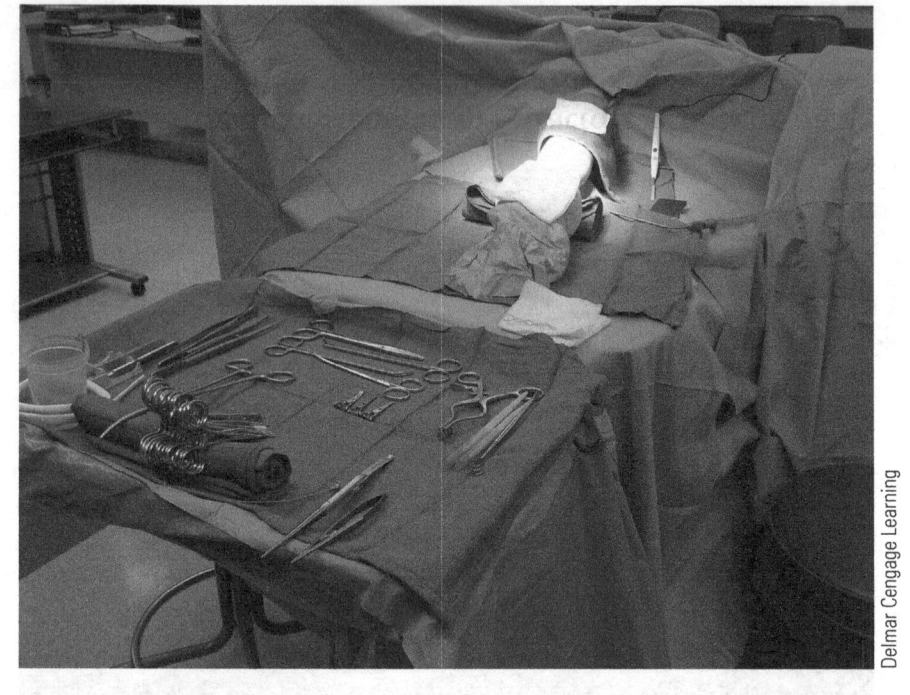

Delmar Cengage Learning

Figure 1-10: Basic Mayo setup for arm/wrist procedures

Figure 1-11 presents a basic Mayo setup for arm/hand/wrist procedures. Instrumentation will be adjusted accordingly. This shows the Mayo setup with the back table pulled up to the sterile field.

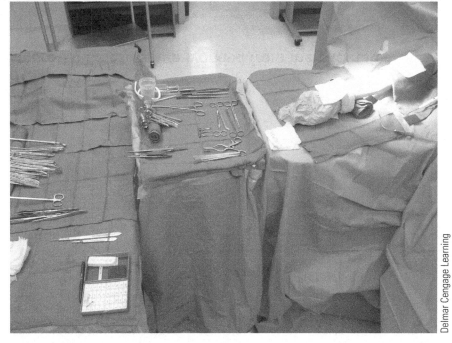

Figure 1-11: Basic Mayo setup for arm/hand/wrist procedure

Figure 1-12 shows a basic setup working from the back table. This layout may be utilized for urology, gynecology, or some orthopedic procedures. The instrumentation would be changed accordingly. This layout is utilized depending on the site of surgery and when there is limited space or no need for a traditional Mayo stand.

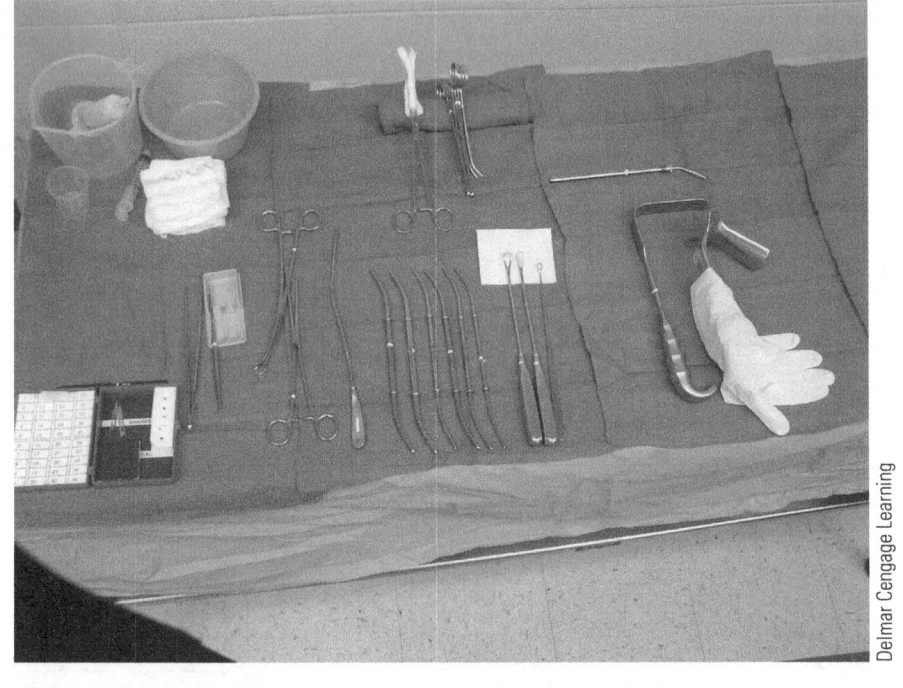

Delmar Cengage Learning

Figure 1-12: Basic setup working from the back table

Conclusion

There are many different variations and techniques for setting up your Mayo stand and back table for different procedures. New or inexperienced scrub personnel will need to find a method they are most comfortable with and that will facilitate the setup and passing of instruments and supplies in the most efficient way during the procedure. Depending on the specialty, there is not always a need for the traditional Mayo stand setup. In some situations, a back table setup will be utilized for instrumentation and supplies without a Mayo setup. This may be done in such cases as cystoscopy, OB/GYN procedures, and hand, wrist, or arm procedures.

Scrub persons will want the Mayo stand setup and/or the back table setup to be organized so that they can reach all instrumentation and supplies. The most commonly used items are traditionally placed on the Mayo stand, whereas the less commonly used items are left on the back table. Instrumentation and supplies must be organized so the surgical count can be performed at the appropriate times. The scrub person will need to multitask at different times during the procedure, so he or she will need to be able to see and reach all instrumentation and supplies.

Having an organized setup will be more beneficial to the patient, as it enables the scrub person to meet the needs of the surgeon and expedite the timely and efficient passing of instruments and supplies. It also decreases the risk of losing an item and facilitates the transition when a team member needs to be relieved during a procedure.

Every scrub person should find his or her own method of setting up the sterile field. In doing so, remember that most facilities have standard protocol that must be followed. Also keep in mind the layout of the OR, the surgeon's preference, and basic technique.

Personal Notes

Chapter 2

General Surgery

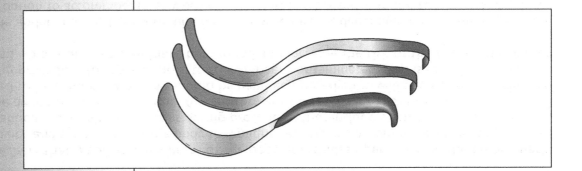

Introduction

General surgery is a specialty that involves many areas of the body. It includes operations on the breast, neck, abdomen, abdominal cavity, and other areas of the body that might have lesions or tumors. It includes operations on the contents of the abdominal cavity. When considering procedures that include operating on the intestines, it is very important to be aware of bowel technique. Any instruments that come into contact with the mucosa of the bowel are considered to be contaminated and should be handled properly. You will need to have additional clean instruments for the procedure to replace those that have been contaminated. This is especially important for closure of the wound, so as not to contaminate the wound and increase the risk of the patient getting an infection.

Procedures done in the abdominal cavity may require a variety of retractors, depending on the surgeon and the need for exposure. One option to accommodate easy access to the larger retractors is to utilize a second Mayo tray setup or a small back table for the larger instruments so that they do not clutter the primary Mayo tray. You can prepare the second Mayo tray with clamps and retractors that are used only occasionally during the procedure.

Your primary Mayo tray should contain the most commonly used instruments for the procedure, organized so that you can easily obtain them to facilitate the procedure and the surgeon's needs.

Considerations for general surgery procedures may include:

- Moistened retractors for protection of organs/tissue.
- Lap rings on sponges.
- Sponges may be weighed to calculate blood loss.
- The length and size of instruments will vary according to procedure and patient.
- If utilizing abdominal and rectal combination setup, take extra care not to cross-contaminate or confuse counts.
- Fiberoptic-lighted cautery and retractors may be used on large abdominal procedures.

List of Procedures

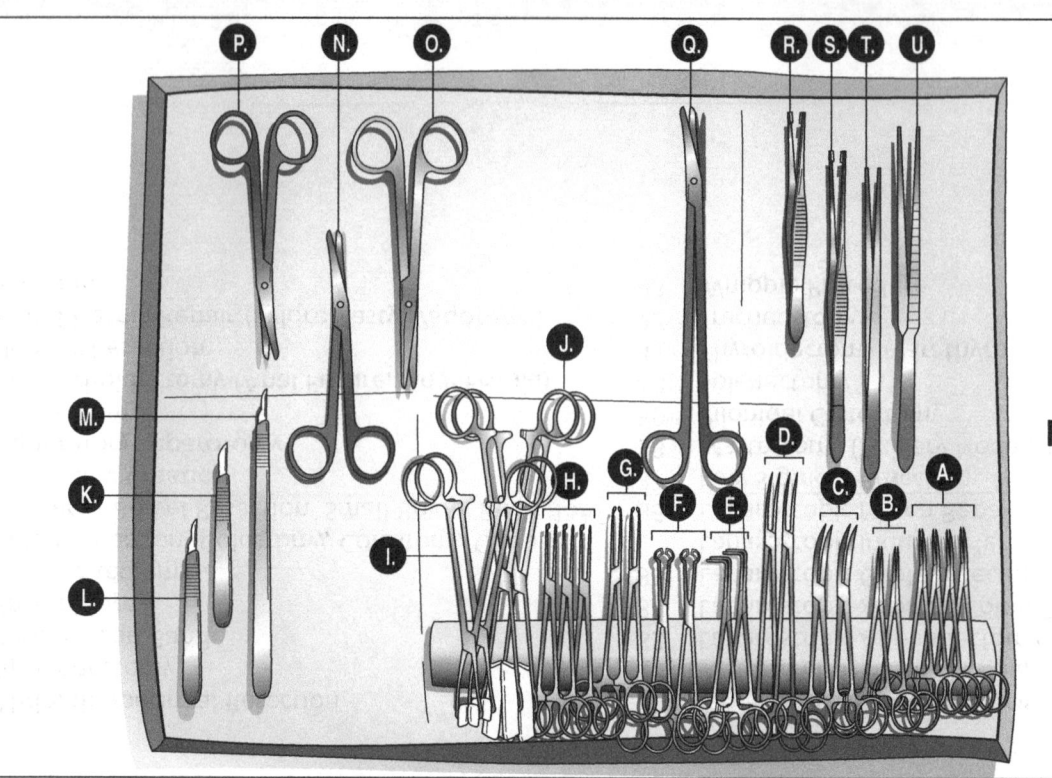

**Primary Setup
First Mayo Tray**

Figure 2-1: Instruments used in an exploratory laparotomy

CLAMPS:

A   curved hemostat
B   straight hemostat
C   Kelly
D   Vanderbilt or Schnidt tonsil artery forces
E   right angle
F   Babcock
G   Allis
H   straight Ochsner
I   curved Ochsner with dissector sponges
J   sponge forceps with 4 × 4 sponges

KNIVES/SCALPELS:

K   #3 handle with 10 blade
L   #3 handle with 15 blade
M   #3 long handle with 15 blade

SCISSORS:

N   curved Mayo
O   straight Mayo
P   regular Metzenbaum
Q   long Metzenbaum

FORCEPS:

R   regular Brown multi-tooth
S   long Brown multi-tooth
T   long smooth
U   DeBakey

Key to Accompany Figure 2-1: Instruments—used in an exploratory laparotomy (Primary Mayo Tray)

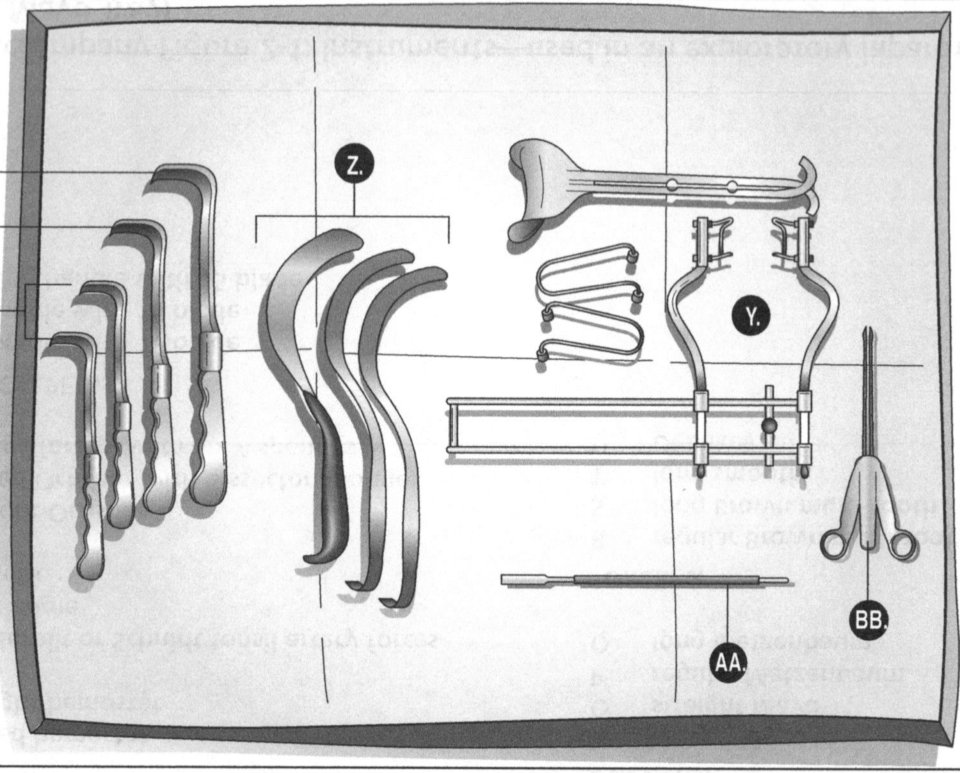
X.
W.
V.
Z.
Y.
AA.
BB.
Second Mayo
Tray

Delmar Cengage Learning

Figure 2-1: Instruments used in an exploratory laparotomy

RETRACTORS:

V   small Richardson
W   medium Richardson
X   large Richardson
Y   Balfour with blades
Z   Deavers

MISCELLANEOUS:

AA   bovie extension
BB   hemoclips

Key to Accompany Figure 2-1: Instruments used in an exploratory laparotomy (Secondary Mayo Tray)

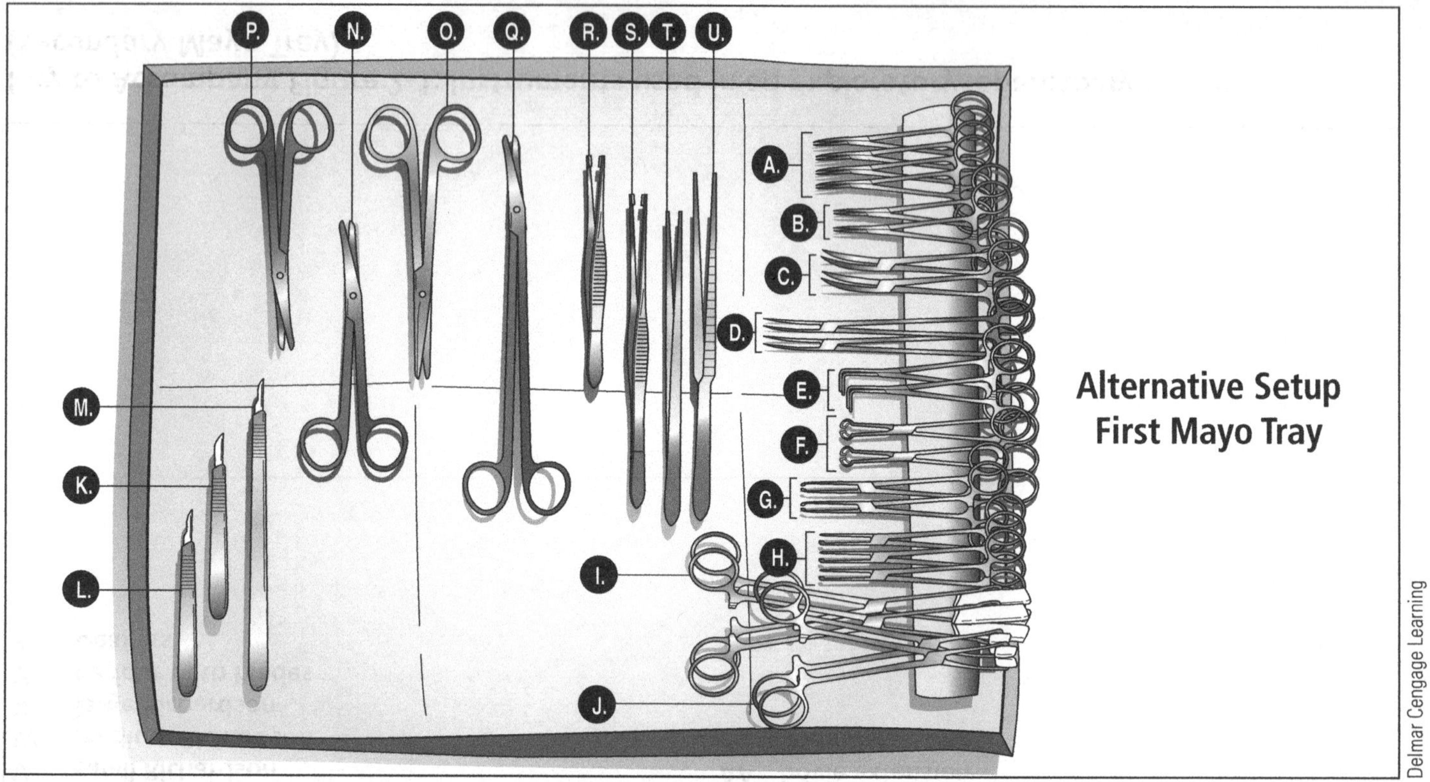
P.
N.
O.
Q.
R.
S.
T.
U.
A.
B.
C.
D.
E.
F.
G.
H.
I.
J.
M.
K.
L.
Alternative Setup
First Mayo Tray
Delmar Cengage Learning

Figure 2-1: Instruments used in an exploratory laparotomy

CLAMPS:

A   curved hemostat
B   straight hemostat
C   Kelly
D   Vanderbilt or Schnidt
E   right angle
F   Babcock
G   Allis
H   straight Ochsner
I   sponge forceps with 4 × 4 sponges
J   curved Ochsner with dissector sponges

KNIVES/SCALPELS:

K   #3 handle with 10 blade
L   #3 handle with 15 blade
M   #3 long handle with 15 blade

SCISSORS:

N   curved Mayo
O   straight Mayo
P   regular Metzenbaum
Q   long Metzenbaum

FORCEPS:

R   regular Brown multi-tooth
S   long Brown multi-tooth
T   long smooth
U   DeBakey

Key to Accompany Figure 2-1: Instruments used in an exploratory laparotomy (alternative setup for Primary Mayo Tray)

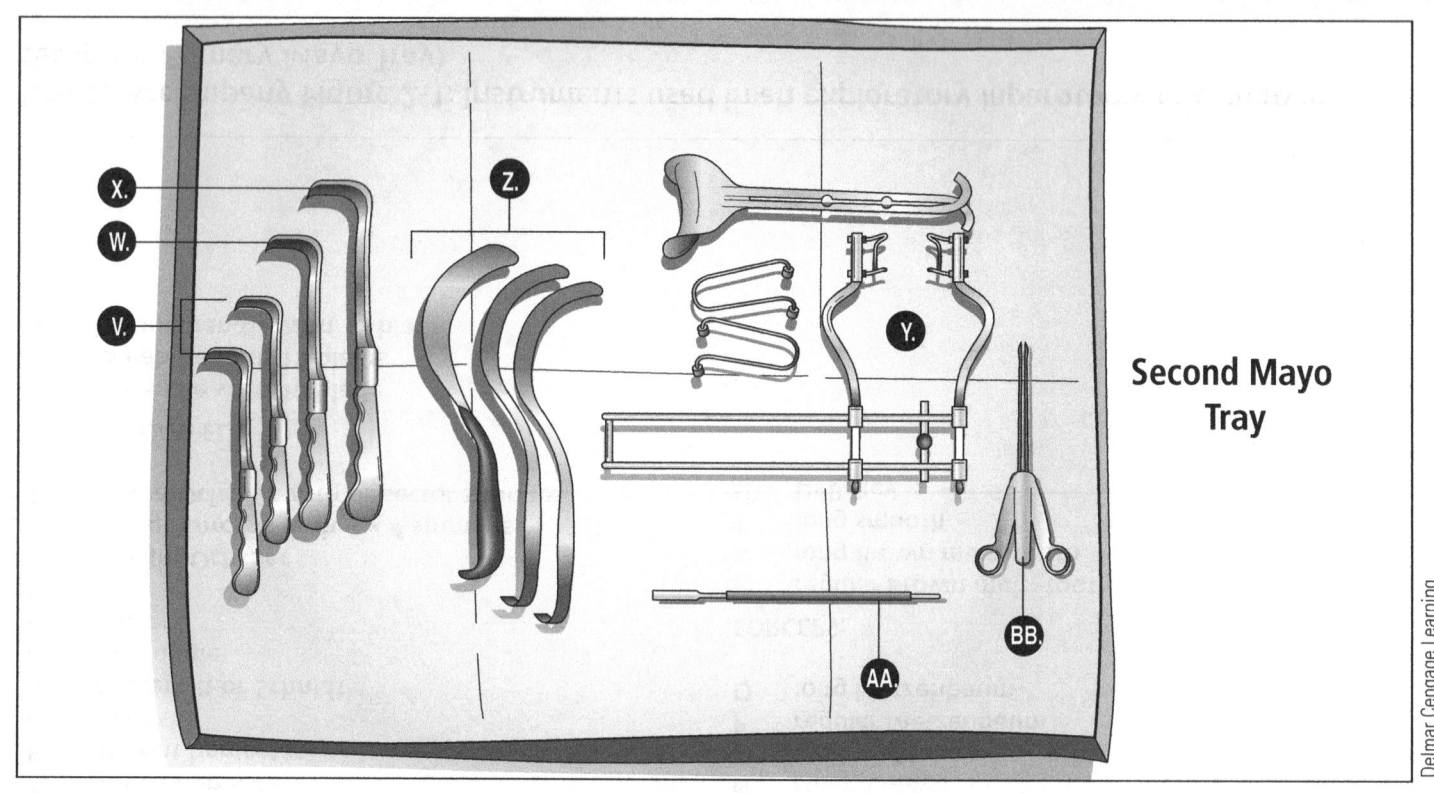

Figure 2-1: Instruments used in an exploratory laparotomy

Second Mayo Tray

RETRACTORS:

V   small Richardson
W   medium Richardson
X   large Richardson
Y   Balfour with blades
Z   Deavers

MISCELLANEOUS:

AA   bovie extension
BB   hemoclips

Key to Accompany Figure 2-1: Instruments used in an exploratory laparotomy (Secondary Mayo Tray)

Delmar Cengage Learning

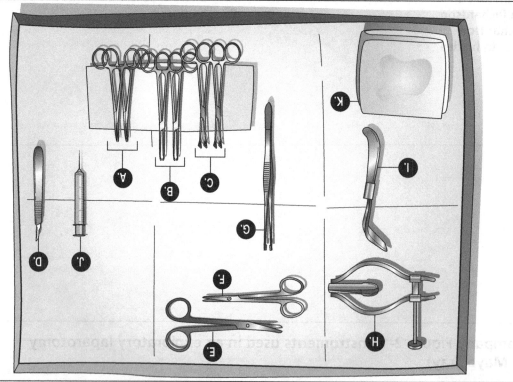

Figure 2-2: Instruments used in a hemorrhoidectomy

CLAMPS:

A   curved hemostat
B   Allis
C   Pennington

KNIVES/SCALPELS:

D   #3 handle with 15 blade

SCISSORS:

E   Metzenbaum (short)
F   straight Mayo

FORCEPS:

G   multi-tooth

RETRACTORS:

H   self-retaining rectal
I   handheld rectal

MISCELLANEOUS:

J   local anesthetic loaded into syringe with
     local injection needle
K   lubricant

Key to Accompany Figure 2-2: Instruments used in a hemorrhoidectomy

Abdominoperineal Resection Setup

Core: General	Level III

Clamps	Knives/Scalpels	Scissors	Forceps	Retractors	Miscellaneous	Notes
• 4 curved mosquito • 6 curved hemostat • 2 straight hemostat • 2 Kelly • 2 Vanderbilt or Schnidt artery forceps • 4 right angle • 2 Babcock • 3 Allis • 3 straight Ochsner • 2 curved Ochsner with dissector sponges • 2 sponge forceps with 4 × 4 sponges • 2 curved intestinal clamps • 2 straight intestinal clamps • 1 right angle intestinal clamp • 2 angled intestinal clamps • 1 J-shaped intestinal clamp	• #4 handle with 20 blade • #3 handle with 10 blade • #3 handle with 15 blade	• regular and long Metzenbaum • straight and curved Mayo	• regular and long Brown multi-tooth • long smooth forceps • 2 pair DeBakey	• 2 small Richardson • 3 Deaver (small, medium, and wide) • 1 large Richardson • Balfour retractor and blades	• sizers • cautery extension • hemoclips • Yankeur • Poole suction and guard	1. Some surgeons use a large self-retaining retractor such as a Bookwalter and blades or Thompson retractor. 2. Because of the nature of this procedure, you will need a Mayo setup for the abdominal portion of the procedure and a back table setup for the lower access. 3. Because of the nature of this procedure, you will need additional instruments or Mayo with clean instruments for closing. 4. Members working below on perineal area need to change gown and gloves prior to closing. 5. Isolate dirty

Back Table Setup for Abdominoperineal Resection

Clamps	Knives/Scalpels	Scissors	Forceps	Retractors	Notes
• 4 curved hemostats • 4 Allis • 2 Babcock • 2 right angles • 2 straight Ochsner	• #3 handle with 10 blade	• Metzenbaum • curved Mayo • straight Mayo	• Brown multi-tooth	• 2 small Richardson • 2 narrow Deaver	1. Have stapling cart/supplies ready in room. 2. May have 2 separate counts.

Appendectomy Setup

Core: General	Level I

Clamps	Knives/Scalpels	Scissors	Forceps	Retractors	Miscellaneous	Notes
• 4 curved hemostat • 3 straight hemostat • 2 Kelly • 2 Allis • 3 Babcock • 2 right angles • 2 straight Ochsner • 2 curved Ochsner with dissector • 1 sponge forceps with 4 × 4 sponge	• #3 handle with 10 blade • #3 handle with 15 blade	• Metzenbaum • straight and curved Mayo	• 2 pair DeBakey • Brown multi-tooth • smooth forceps	• 2 small Richardson • appendectomy retractors • 2 medium Gelpi	• medium hemoclips	1. As some surgeons choose to take a culture upon entering the peritoneal cavity, you may need a culture tube on your Mayo tray. 2. Isolate specimens and instruments coming in contact with inside of specimen. 3. Irrigation with antibiotic solution often used. 4. May need drain.

Bariatric Lap Band

Core: General	Level II

Clamps	Knives/Scalpels	Scissors	Forceps	Retractors	Miscellaneous	Notes
• 2 curved hemostats • 2 straight Ochsners • 2 Kelly	• #3 handle with 11 blade	• straight Mayo • Endo	• DeBakey • Ferguson • Adson single tooth	• 2 medium Richardsons • Endo liver	• Endo graspers • Lap Band • Band introducer • Band passer • 20 mL syringe • Knot pusher • 10 mm 0-degree scope • 30-degree scope • Gas cord • Light cord • Camera • Anti-fog	1. Procedure is performed on obese patients, so will need appropriate table and positioning devices.

Breast Biopsy Setup

Core: General	Level I

Clamps	Knives/Scalpels	Scissors	Forceps	Retractors	Miscellaneous	Notes
• 4 curved hemostat • 2 Allis • 2 Lahey • 2 right angle	• 2 #3 handle with 15 blade	• short and regular Metzenbaums • curved Mayo • straight Mayo	• Brown multi-tooth • 2 pair DeBakey	• 2 Senn • 2 Army–Navy • 2 Richardson • 2 skin hook	• marking pen • cautery needle tip	1. If the procedure is to be done under a local anesthetic, you will need to have the surgeon's preference of medication, syringes, and local injection needles. 2. If procedure is done following a needle localization, the specimen will be sent to Radiology before being sent to Pathology. 3. Mastectomy may be performed following diagnosis. See Mastectomy Setup.

Cholecystectomy Setup

Core: General		Level II

Clamps	Knives/Scalpels	Scissors	Forceps	Retractors	Miscellaneous	Notes
• 4 curved hemostat • 2 straight hemostat • 2 Vanderbilt • 2 Kelly • 2 Allis • 2 right angle • 3 straight Ochsner • 1 catheter clamp • 1 sponge forceps with 4 × 4 sponge • 2 curved Ochsner with dissectors • 2 long Kelly	• 2 #3 handle with 10 blade • #3 long handle with 15 blade	• regular and long Metzenbaum • curved and straight Mayo	• regular smooth forceps • regular Brown multi-tooth • long Brown multi-tooth • regular DeBakey • Ferris-Smith	• 2 small Richardson	• medium hemoclips	1. Have easily accessible on the back table: 2 Harrington retractors, Deaver retractors, cholangiogram supplies, and gallbladder instruments if you have to perform a common bile duct exploration (CBDE). 2. If a CBDE is done, you will need to add gallbladder scoops, Bakes dilators, Potts–Smith scissors, Randall stone forceps, and a scope.

Colon Resection Setup

Core: General		Level II

Clamps	Knives/Scalpels	Scissors	Forceps	Retractors	Notes	
• 6 curved hemostat • 2 straight hemostat • 2 Kelly • 2 Vanderbilt • 2 right angle • 2 Babcock • 3 regular Allis • 2 long Allis • 3 straight Ochsner • 2 curved Ochsner with dissector sponges • 2 sponge forceps with 4 × 4 sponges • 2 curved non-crushing gastro-intestinal clamps • 2 angled non-crushing gastro-intestinal clamps • 2 straight non-crushing gastro-intestinal clamps	• #3 handle with 10 blade • #3 long handle with 15 blade • #4 handle with 20 blade	• curved Mayo • straight Mayo • regular and long Metzenbaum	• long Russian • regular and long Brown multi-tooth • long smooth forceps • 2 pair of DeBakey • Ferris-Smith	• 2 small, 1 medium, and 1 large Richardson • 2 Deaver	1. May also need long or wide Deaver retractors. 2. Have Balfour retractor available upon opening peritoneum. 3. Upon wound closure, you will need to have available on another Mayo or ready to replace on working Mayo: clean suture scissors, Metzenbaum scissors, Brown multi-tooth forceps, and sutures for closing.	4. May need to change gown/gloves. 5. Mayo setup may also be used for: small bowel resection, large bowel resection, colostomy, and colostomy closure.

Colostomy Creation Setup

Core: General	Level II

Clamps	Knives/Scalpels	Scissors	Forceps	Retractors	Miscellaneous	Notes
• 4 curved hemostats • 2 straight hemostats • 2 Kelly • 2 right angle • 2 Babcocks • 4 Crile	• #3 handle with 10 blade • #3 handle with 15 blade	• Metzenbaum • curved Mayo • straight Mayo	• 2 DeBakey • Brown multi-tooth • Ferguson	• 2 Army–Navy • 2 small Richardson	• medium hemoclip appliers • GI linear staplers	1. Balfour self-retaining retractor may be used. 2. Bowel technique must be followed. 3. Colostomy supplies must be available: rod, drainage bag, suture, etc.

Exploratory Laparotomy Setup

Core: General	Level II

Clamps	Knives/Scalpels	Scissors	Forceps	Retractors	Miscellaneous	Notes
• 4 curved hemostat • 2 straight hemostat • 2 Kelly • 2 Vanderbilt • 2 right angle • 2 Babcock • 2 Allis • 3 straight Ochsner • 2 curved Ochsner with dissector sponges • 2 sponge forceps with 4 × 4 sponges	• #3 with 10 blade • #3 handle with 15 blade • #3 long handle with 15 blade	• curved Mayo • straight Mayo • regular and long Metzenbaum	• regular and long Brown multi-tooth • long smooth forceps • 2 pair of DeBakey • Ferris-Smith	• 2 small, 1 medium, and 1 large Richardson • 1 Balfour with blades • 3 Deaver	• bovie extension • hemoclips	1. Have stapling instruments/ supplies available. 2. A second Mayo setup may be used for holding the retractors. 3. If procedure turns into colon resection, you may need additional gastrointestinal instruments. Bowel technique must be followed.

Gastrectomy Setup

Core: General	Level II

Clamps	Knives/Scalpels	Scissors	Forceps	Retractors	Miscellaneous
• 4 curved mosquito • 4 curved hemostat • 2 straight hemostat • 2 Kelly • 2 Vanderbilt • 2 right angle • 2 regular and 2 long Babcock • 4 regular and 2 long Allis • 3 straight Ochsner • 2 curved Ochsner with dissector • 2 sponge forceps with 4 × 4 sponges • 2 Doyen intestinal forceps	• #4 handle with 20 blade • #3 handle with 10 blade • #3 long handle with 15 blade	• regular and long Metzenbaum • curved and straight Mayo	• regular and long Brown multi-tooth • long smooth • 2 pair DeBakey • Ferris-Smith	• 2 small Richardson • 1 medium Richardson • Balfour with blade • 3 Deaver (narrow, medium, and wide) • 2 Harrington	• hemoclip applicators and clips. • medium and large blunt nerve hook • Penrose drain

Hemorrhoidectomy Setup

Core: General	Level I

Clamps	Knives/Scalpels	Scissors	Forceps	Retractors	Miscellaneous	Notes
• 2 curved hemostat • 2 Allis • 2 Pennington	• #3 handle with 15 blade	• Metzenbaum • straight Mayo • rectal	• multi-tooth	• self-retaining rectal • handheld rectal	• Local anesthetic loaded into syringe with local injection needle • Water-soluble lubricant or Betadine • Probe groove director	1. May use anoscope, which would need to be set up in a ring basin or on a separate small Mayo tray. 2. This Mayo setup may also be used for: anal fissure and anal fistula.

Hepatic Resection Setup

Core: General	Level II

Clamps	Knives/Scalpels	Scissors	Forceps	Miscellaneous	Notes
• 6 curved hemostat • 2 straight hemostat • 2 Kelly • 4 Vanderbilt • 4 right angle • 4 Crile • 2 Babcock • 2 Allis • 3 straight Ochsner • 2 curved Ochsner loaded with dissectors • 2 sponge forceps with 4 × 4 sponges • 2 curved Doyen intestinal clamps • 2 straight Doyen intestinal clamps • 2 DeBakey non-crushing vascular clamps • 2 right angle vascular clamps	• #4 handle with 20 blade • #3 handle with 10 blade • #3 long handle with 15 blade	• regular and long Metzenbaum • curved and straight Mayo	• regular and long Brown multi-tooth • long smooth forceps • 2 pair DeBakey • long Russian	• hemoclip applicator and clips • cautery extension 2. For a thoraco-abdominal approach, you would need to add the following to the Mayo tray: • Finochietto rib spreader • Duval–Crile lung clamp • Alexander costal periosteotome • Alexander rib raspatory • Bailey rib approximator • wire cutters/scissors	1. Because of the number of retractors that may be used during this procedure, one option is to set up a second Mayo tray for retractors. It would include: Retractors: • 2 small, 2 medium, and 1 large Richardson • narrow, medium, and wide Deaver • extra-long or wide Deaver • 2 Harrington • self-retaining retractor such as Balfour with blades

Hiatal Hernia Repair Setup

Core: General	Level II

Clamps	Knives/Scalpels	Scissors	Forceps	Retractors	Miscellaneous	Notes
• 4 curved mosquito • 6 curved hemostat • 2 straight hemostat • 4 Kelly • 4 Vanderbilt or Crile • 2 regular right angle • 2 long right angle • 2 Babcock • 2 Allis • 3 straight Ochsner • 2 curved Ochsner loaded with dissector sponges • 2 sponge forceps with 4 × 4 sponges • 2 curved gastrointestinal clamps	• #4 handle with 20 blade • #3 handle with 10 blade • #3 long handle with 15 blade	• regular and long Metzenbaum • curved and straight Mayo	• regular and long Brown multi-tooth • long smooth • 2 pair long DeBakey • Ferris-Smith	• large self-retaining retractor such as Balfour and/or Bookwalter • 2 small, 2 medium, and 1 large Richardson • various Deavers • 2 Harrington • 2 malleable	• Cautery extension • blunt nerve hook • hemoclip applicators • Penrose drain • esophageal dilators	1. Some may choose to use an additional Mayo tray to hold the retractors. 2. Mayo setup may also be used for: vagotomy and pyloroplasty.

Ileostomy Setup

Core: General	Level II

Clamps	Knives/Scalpels	Scissors	Forceps	Retractors	Miscellaneous	Notes
• 4 curved hemostats • 2 straight hemostats • 4 Kelly • 2 Crile • 2 right angle • 2 Babcock • 2 Allis • 2 sponge sticks loaded with 4 × 4 sponges • 2 curved Ochsners	• #3 handle with 10 blade • #3 handle with 15 blade	• Metzenbaum • straight Mayo • curved Mayo • long Metzenbaum	• Brown multi-tooth • 2 pair DeBakey • smooth	• 2 small Richardsons • 2 Army–Navy • Second Mayo setup may include larger retractors, such as: • 2 Deavers • 2 Harrington • 1 body wall • 2 medium Richardson • 1 Balfour	• GI linear staplers • marking pen • hemoclip appliers, small and medium	1. GI clamps may very according to surgeon's preference. 2. Colostomy may be temporary or permanent. 3. Bowel technique should be followed. 4. Have ostomy supplies available: rod, drainage bag, suture, etc.

Inguinal Hernia Repair Setup

Core: General	Level I

Clamps	Knives/Scalpels	Scissors	Forceps	Retractors	Miscellaneous	Notes
• 4 curved hemostat • 2 straight hemostat • 2 Kelly • 2 right angle • 1 Babcock • 2 Allis • 1 straight Ochsner • 1 curved Ochsner with dissector • 1 sponge forceps with 4 × 4 sponge	• #3 handle with 10 blade • #3 handle with 15 blade	• regular and short Metzenbaum • curved and straight Mayo	• multi-tooth • smooth forceps • 2 pair DeBakey	• 2 small Richardson • 1 medium Richardson • 2 Gelpi or other self-retaining	• hemoclips • Penrose drain (for male patients)	1. Mayo setup may also be used for: ventral hernia repair, incisional hernia repair, and umbilical hernia repair. 2. May inject local anesthetic for post-op pain, so will need syringe, hypodermic needle, and medication.

Laparoscopic Appendectomy Setup

Core: General	Level II

(Because of the specific instrumentation for laparoscopy procedures, you will not need to categorize these instruments.)

		Miscellaneous	Notes
• 1 Allis clamp • 2 curved hemo-stat clamps • 2 towel clips • #3 knife handle with 15 blade • straight Mayo scissors • Brown multi-tooth forceps • single-tooth Adson forceps • 5 mm trocar • 10 mm trocar • #12 trocar • Verres needle • reducer • anti-fog • 2 laparoscopic graspers • laparoscopic scissors	• laparoscopic dissector • probe • camera • scope • light cord	• May need endo sta-pling device	1. Always have an open setup available.

Laparoscopic-Assisted Colon Resection Setup

Core: General	Level III

Clamps	Knives/Scalpels	Scissors	Forceps	Retractors	Miscellaneous	Notes
• 4 curved hemostats • 2 straight hemostats • 2 Kelly • 2 curved GI clamps • 2 angled GI clamps • endo right angle • endo grasper • endo Babcock	• #3 handle with 15 blade • #3 handle with 10 blade	• Metzenbaum • straight Mayo • endo scissors	• Brown multi-tooth • 2 pair DeBakey	• 2 small Richardson • endo	• endo cautery and suction • 10 mm trocar • 12 mm Hasson trocar • 2 12 mm trocar • 5 mm port • endo clips • endo linear staplers • GI linear staplers • camera and cord • light source cord • anti-fog • laparoscopic dissector • Verres needle • insufflator needle and tubing	1. Colon dissection may be performed laparoscopically and then mini-lap performed for removal of specimen and anastomosis. 2. Have open setup available.

Laparoscopic Cholecystectomy Setup

Core: General	Level II

(Because of the specific instrumentation for laparoscopy procedures, you will not need to categorize these instruments.)

		Notes
• 2 laparoscopic graspers • 1 laparoscopic dissector • probe • 2 towel clips • laparoscopic scissors • 1 large gallbladder grasper • 2 Allis clamps • 2 curved hemostat clamps • 2 Kelly clamps • scope • camera • light cord • #3 knife handle with 15 blade • straight Mayo scissors	• Brown multi-tooth forceps • single-tooth Adson forceps • 2 Hasson "S" retractors • 2 Army–Navy retractors • 2 5 mm trocars • 2 10 mm trocars • medium/large ligaclips • reducers • Verres needle • anti-fog	1. Cholangiogram kit includes catheter and syringes loaded with dye and saline with all air bubbles removed. 2. Always have open setup available. 3. May need endo catch for specimen.

Laparoscopic Inguinal Hernia Repair Setup

Core: General	Level II

(Because of the specific instrumentation for laparoscopy procedures, you will not need to categorize these instruments.)

		Notes
• 2 laparoscopic dissectors • Kelly clamps • 12 mm blunt trocar • 2 5 mm hernia trocar • 1 hernia balloon trocar • 2 Allis clamps • hernia repair staple gun • #3 knife handle with 15 blade • straight Mayo scissors • Brown multi-tooth forceps • single-tooth Adson forceps • Hasson "S" retractor • mesh	• camera • scope • light cord • 2 laparoscopic kitners • anti-fog	1. May need mesh or mesh plug. 2. May need antibiotic irrigation. 3. Have open setup available.

Laparoscopic Nissen Repair Setup

Core: General	Level II

(Because of the specific instrumentation for laparoscopy procedures, you will not need to categorize these instruments.)

		Notes
• 2 laparoscopic graspers • 2 laparoscopic dissectors • laparoscopic scissors • laparoscopic balloon retractor • endo-maxi retractor • 5 10 mm trocar • 5 mm trocar • reducer cap • #3 knife handle with 15 blade • straight Mayo scissors • Brown multi-tooth forceps • Adson single-tooth forceps • camera • scope	• light cord • angle scope • anti-fog	1. You will need some type of knot-pushing suture such as Ethibond (depends on surgeon's preference). 2. Have open setup available.

Low Sigmoid Resection Setup

Core: General	Level II

Clamps	Knives/Scalpels	Scissors	Forceps	Retractors	Notes	
• 4 curved hemostat • 2 straight hemostat • 2 regular and 2 long Kelly • 2 regular and 2 long right angle • 2 regular and 2 long Babcock • 2 regular and 2 long Allis • 3 straight Ochsner • 2 curved Ochsner with dissectors • 2 sponge forceps with 4 × 4 sponges • 1 long-angled non-crushing intestinal clamps • 2 straight and 2 curved non-crushing	• #3 handle with 10 blade • #3 long handle with 15 blade • #4 handle with 20 blade	• regular and long Metzenbaum • straight and curved Mayo	• regular and long Brown multi-tooth • long smooth forceps • 2 pair DeBakey • Russian	• 2 small Richardson • 3 Deaver • 2 Harrington • Balfour with blades • large Richardson • 2 medium Richardson A large type of self-retaining retractor may also be needed.	1. Some people choose to use a separate Mayo tray with the larger retractors so that they are easier accessed during the procedure. 2. Surgeon may perform proctoscopy prior to start of procedure. If so, can set up sterile proctoscope in sterile ring basin.	3. A separate small table may be set up for the lower portion of the procedure with extra gloves, drapes, dilators, stapling devices, lubricant, and so forth. 4. Patient may be in some variation of lithotomy position.

Mastectomy Setup

Core: General	Level II

Clamps	Knives/Scalpels	Scissors	Forceps	Retractors	Miscellaneous	Notes
• 4 curved hemostat • 2 straight hemostat • 2 Kelly • 2 regular and 1 long right angle • 2 Vanderbilt or Crile • 4 Allis • 2 straight Ochsner • 6 breast tenaculum • 6 Lahey • 2 curved Ochsner with dissectors	• #3 handle with 15 blade • #3 handle with 10 blade	• regular and long Metzenbaum • curved and straight Mayo	• 2 pair DeBakey • 1 regular and 1 long Brown multi-tooth • 1 long smooth	• 1 small and 2 medium Richardson	• 4 skin hooks • marking pen • hemoclips • cautery extension	1. Mayo setup may also be used for: lumpectomy and axillary node dissection. 2. If performed immediately following a biopsy, you will need two separate setups to prevent the spread of cancerous cells. 3. Drain may be placed at end of procedure. 4. May change gloves after removal of specimen prior to closing. 5. May need pressure dressing.

Pilonidal Cystectomy Setup

Core: General		Level I

Clamps	Knives/Scalpels	Scissors	Forceps	Miscellaneous	Notes
• 2 curved hemostat • 2 straight hemostat • 1 Kelly • 2 Allis	• #3 handle with 15 blade	• regular and short Metzenbaum • straight and curved Mayo	• regular Brown multi-tooth • regular smooth forceps • Adson with single tooth • 2 small Richardson	• probe and groove • sharp curettes	1. Methylene blue loaded into a syringe with a blunt needle is sometimes used depending on surgeon's preference. 2. May pack wound and leave open. 3. Bulk dressing may be needed.

Splenectomy Setup

Core: General	Level II

Clamps	Knives/Scalpels	Scissors	Forceps	Retractors	Miscellaneous	Notes
• 4 curved hemostat • 2 straight hemostat • 2 Kelly • 2 Vanderbilt • 2 right angle • 2 Babcock • 2 Allis • 3 straight Ochsner • 2 curved Ochsner loaded with dissectors • 2 sponge forceps with 4 × 4 sponges • 2 angled vascular clamps • 2 curved vascular clamps • 2 right angle vascular clamps	• 2 #3 handle with 10 blade • #3 long handle with 15 blade	• regular and long Metzenbaum • curved and straight Mayo	• regular and long Brown multi-tooth • 2 pair DeBakey • Russian • long smooth	• 2 small Richardson	• hemoclips • cautery extensions	1. Some people choose to have a second Mayo with the larger retractors convenient to the primary Mayo for quick access. It would include the following retractors: • 2 Harrington • 3 Deaver • 2 medium Richardson • 1 large Richardson 2. Excessive bleeding may occur.

Thyroidectomy Setup

Core: General	Level II

Clamps	Knives/Scalpels	Scissors	Forceps	Retractors	Miscellaneous	Notes
• 6 mosquito hemostat • 6 curved hemostat • 2 straight hemostat • 2 Kelly • 2 right angle • 4 Allis • 2 curved Ochsner with dissectors • 4 Lahey	• #3 handle with 10 blade • #3 handle with 15 blade	• regular and short Metzenbaum • straight Mayo	• 2 pair medium DeBakey • regular Brown multi-tooth • regular smooth • bipolar	• 2 Army–Navy • 2 small Richardson • 2 skin hook • 2 Gelpi • 2 Green • 2 double-prong skin books • lone star	• marking pen	1. Mayo setup may also be used for: parathyroidectomy. 2. May be performed by general or ENT surgeon. 3. Keep specimens separated. 4. Some surgeons use a free hand tie to mark the neck for the incision line. This is done to create a more precise scar along the creases in the skin along the neck.

Tracheostomy Setup

Core: General	Level II

Clamps	Knives/Scalpels	Scissors	Forceps	Retractors	Miscellaneous	Notes
• 4 curved hemostat • 3 Allis • 2 right angle • 2 straight hemostats	• #3 handle with 15 blade • #3 handle with 11 blade	• Metzenbaum • curved and straight Mayo	• Brown multi-tooth • smooth forceps • Adson with teeth • DeBakey	• 2 Senn • 2 Army–Navy • 2 small Richardson • 2 Gelpi	• trach dilator • trach spreader • trach hook • needle holder loaded with stay suture of surgeon's preference • umbilical tapes • suction catheter • 10 cc syringe • needle tip bovie • syringe and needle loaded with local anesthetic of surgeon's preference • marking pen	1. Have tracheostomy tubes of all sizes available in room for circulator to open when surgeon determines size to be used. This will then go on your Mayo tray. 2. Be sure that the obturator from the trach tubes is sent with the patient after the procedure. 3. Be sure to check the patency of the trach balloon. 4. May be performed on ICU bed. 5. Have headlight available.

Whipple Procedure Setup

Core: General	Level III

Clamps	Knives/Scalpels	Scissors	Forceps	Retractors	Miscellaneous	Notes
• 4 hemostat • 6 curved and 2 straight hemostat • 2 Kelly • 4 Vanderbilt • 4 right angle • 4 Babcock • 2 Allis • 3 straight Ochsner • 2 curved Ochsner loaded with dissectors • 2 sponge forceps with 4 × 4 sponges • 2 curved non-crushing intestinal clamps • 2 straight non-crushing intestinal clamps • 2 Payr • 2 Allen	• #4 handle with 20 blade • #3 handle with 10 blade • #3 handle with 15 blade	• regular and long Metzenbaum • curved and straight Mayo • Potts-Smith	• regular and long Brown multi-tooth • long smooth forceps • 2 pair DeBakey • Russian	• 2 small Richardson • large self-retaining	• hemoclips • cautery extension	1. A second Mayo may be used to accommodate the necessary retractors and stapling equipment. It would include the following retractors: • 2 medium Richardson • 1 large Richardson • 3 Deaver (narrow, medium, wide) • 2 Harrington • Balfour with blades 2. Bowel technique may be required.

Personal Notes

Personal Notes

Chapter 3

Obstetric/ Gynecologic (OB/GYN) Surgery

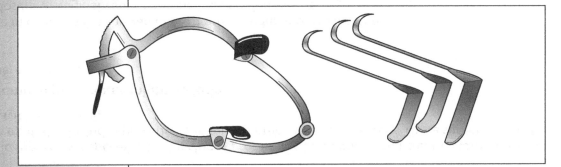

Introduction

Obstetric and gynecologic surgery is a specialty that includes procedures to diagnose and treat conditions of the female reproductive system. It also includes procedures involving pregnancy and delivery. These surgeries may be performed in the pelvic cavity or vaginally.

Considerations for abdominal procedures might include:

- Check sterilization operative consent.
- Moist packing laps.
- Sponge sticks.
- Instruments that come in contact with the vaginal cuff are considered contaminated.
- Counts are taken at closure of vaginal vault, peritoneum, and skin closure.

Considerations for cesarean section may include:

- Bulb syringes are used.
- Additional counts are performed at closure of uterus.

Considerations for vaginal or perineal procedures include:

- Sponges on sponge forceps are opened lengthwise.
- Vaginal packs are used and must be counted properly.
- Telfa may be used for scrapings/specimens.

Prior to most OB/GYN, the bladder should be drained to protect it from injury. An indwelling catheter is often left in place for abdominal OB/GYN procedures.

If multiple procedures are to be performed, the diagnostic portion is done first. If combination vaginal/abdominal procedures are to be performed, the abdominal portion is done first.

Facilities may utilize specialty trays designed for specific cases due to the nature of instrumentation. They may be all inclusive or used in conjunction with basic instrumentation sets with the addition of specialty clamps, and so forth.

List of Procedures

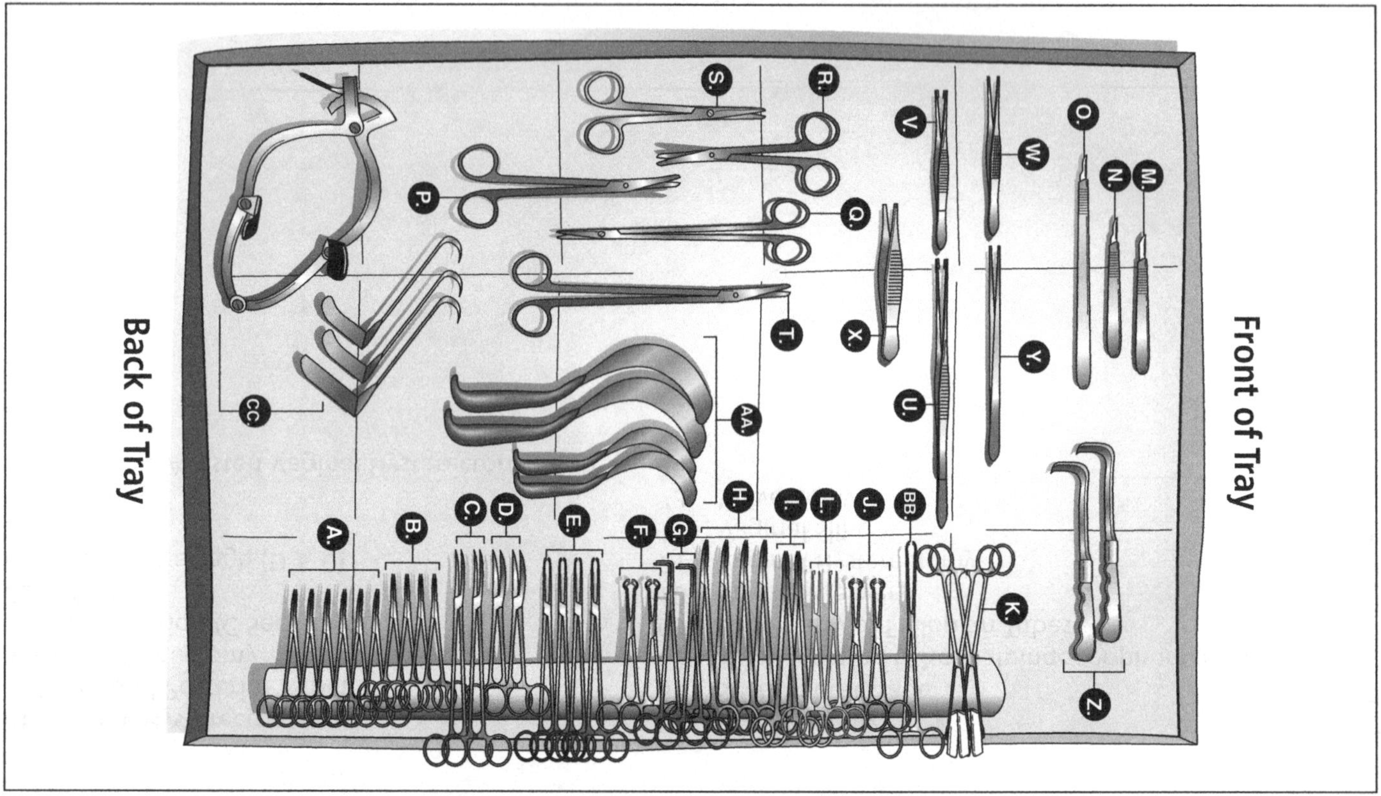

Figure 3-1: Instruments used in an abdominal hysterectomy

CLAMPS:

A   curved hemostat
B   straight hemostat
C   Vanderbilt or Crile
D   Kelly
E   long Allis
F   Babcock
G   long right angle
H   curved Heaney
I   straight Heaney
J   straight Ochsner
K   sponge forceps with 4 × 4 sponges
L   Lahey

KNIVES/SCALPELS:

M   #3 handle with 10 blade
N   #3 handle with 15 blade
O   #3 long handle with 15 blade

SCISSORS:

P   regular Metzenbaum
Q   long Metzenbaum

R   curved Mayo
S   straight Mayo
T   Jorgenson

FORCEPS:

U   long Brown multi-tooth
V   regular Brown multi-tooth
W   Bonney
X   Ferris–Smith
Y   long smooth

RETRACTORS:

Z   small Richardson
AA   Deaver

MISCELLANEOUS:

BB   tenaculum
CC   O'Sullivan–O'Connor self-retaining retractor with bladder blade

Key to Accompany Figure 3-1: Instruments used in an abdominal hysterectomy

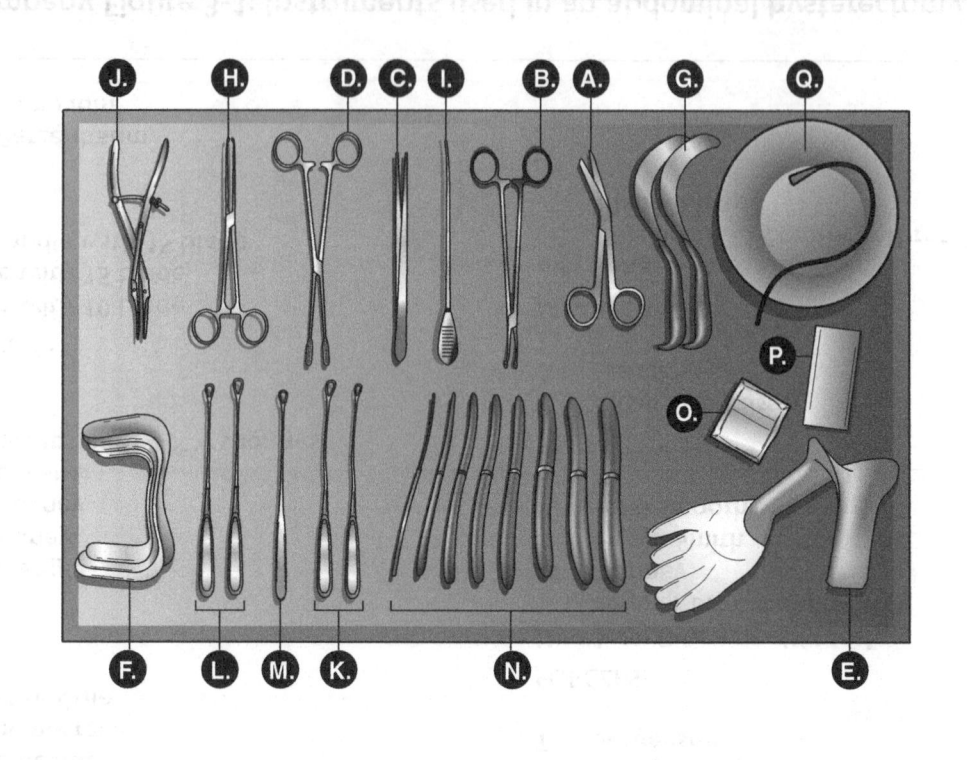

Figure 3-2: Instruments used in a Dilation & Curettage (D & C)

SCISSORS:

A   bandage scissors

FORCEPS:

B   Gaylor dressing
C   long smooth
D   polyp

RETRACTORS:

E   weighted vaginal speculum with glove stretched on the end
F   Sims
G   small Deaver

MISCELLANEOUS:

H   tenaculum
I   uterine sounds
J   Goodell dilators
K   small and medium Sims sharp curettes
L   small and medium Thomas curettes
M   Heaney curette
N   Hegar dilators
O   K-Y jelly
P   Telfa
Q   small basin with red rubber catheter

Key to Accompany Figure 3-2: Instruments used in a Dilation & Curettage (D & C)

Abdominal Hysterectomy Setup

Core: OB/GYN	Level II

Clamps	Knives/Scalpels	Scissors	Forceps	Retractors	Miscellaneous	Notes
• 6 curved hemostat • 4 straight hemostat • 2 Vanderbilt or Crile • 2 Kelly • 4 long Allis • 2 Babcock • 2 long right angle • 4 curved Heaney • 2 straight Heaney • 2 straight Ochsner • Sponge forceps with 4 × 4 sponges • 2 Lahey	• #3 handle with 10 blade • #3 long handle with 15 blade	• regular and long Metzenbaum • curved and straight Mayo • Jorgenson	• long and regular Brown multi-tooth • Bonney • Ferris-Smith • long smooth	• 2 small Richardson • 2 Deaver	• tenaculum	1. Have ready the O'Sullivan-O'Connor self-retaining retractor with bladder blade.

Anterior and Posterior Repair Setup

Core: OB/GYN	Level I

Clamps	Knives/Scalpels	Scissors	Forceps	Retractors	Miscellaneous	Notes
• 6 curved hemostat • 6 Allis • 2 sponge forceps with 4 × 4 sponges	• #3 handle with 15 blade	• Metzenbaum • curved and straight Mayo	• Brown multi-tooth • long smooth	• Auvard weighted vaginal speculum with glove stretched over the end • 2 Sims • 2 small Deaver	• tenaculum	1. Most people do not use a Mayo tray; they prepare a back table to work from because of the position of the patient and limited amount of room.

Bartholin Cystectomy Setup

Core: OB/GYN	Level I

Clamps	Knives/Scalpels	Scissors	Forceps	Retractors	Miscellaneous	Notes
• 4 Allis • 4 Crile • 2 straight Ochsners	• #3 handle with 15 blade • #3 handle with 11 blade	• straight Mayo • curved Mayo • Metzenbaum	• single tooth • smooth	• Heaney	• culture tube	1. Setup may be on backtable instead of Mayo tray. 2. Patient in lithotomy position. 3. May need catheter.

Cesarean Section (C-Section) Setup

Core: OB/GYN	Level II

Clamps	Knives/Scalpels	Scissors	Forceps	Retractors	Miscellaneous
• 4 curved hemostat • 4 Pennington • 4 sponge forceps • 2 straight Ochsner • 2 Allis	• #3 handle with 10 blade • #3 handle with 15 blade • #4 handle with 20 blade	• Metzenbaum • straight and curved Mayo • bandage scissors	• Brown multi-tooth • Bonney • Ferris–Smith	• Delee • 2 small and 1 medium Richardson	• 2 cord blood tubes • 1 cord clamp • bulb syringe

Cone Biopsy Back Table Setup

Core: OB/GYN	Level I

Clamps	Knives/Scalpels	Scissors	Forceps	Retractors	Miscellaneous	Notes
• 2 straight hemostat	• #3 long handle with 11 blade	• curved Mayo	• smooth	• vaginal speculum • right angle • Heaney • small Deaver	• Heaney endo-metrial curette • tenaculum	1. Telfa will be used for specimen. 2. This procedure could be performed with cryosurgery or electrocautery surgery. 3. D & C setup also used. 4. May need Lugol's Solution on sponge stick with 4 × 4 sponge. 5. May use a traction suture.

Dilation & Curettage (D&C) Back Table Setup

Core: OB/GYN	Level I

Scissors	Forceps	Retractors	Miscellaneous	Notes
• bandage scissors	• Gaylor dressing • long smooth • polyp	• Auvard weighted vaginal speculum with glove stretched on the end • 2 Sims • 2 small Deaver	• tenaculum • uterine sound • Goodell dilators • small and medium Sims sharp curettes • small and medium Thomas curettes • Heaney curette • Hegar dilators • K-Y jelly • Telfa • small basin with red rubber catheter • May need Pratt or Hank dilators	1. For this Setup, most people choose to work from their back table instead of using a Mayo tray. 2. You may have two (endometrial and endocervical) specimens, which must remain separated.

Hysteroscopy Back Table Setup

Core: OB/GYN	Level I

Miscellaneous
• weighted speculum • tenaculum • uterine sound • Hegar or Hank dilators • hysteroscope • obturator • sheath • hysteroscopic scissors • hysteroscopic biopsy forceps: Tru-cut and round • hysteroscopic grasping forceps • K-Y jelly • slides • tubing • metal connector/piece • 60 mL syringe

Laparoscopy Setup

Core: OB/GYN	Level II

Scissors	Knives/Scalpels	Forceps	Retractors	Miscellaneous	Notes
• laparoscopic	• #3 handle with 15 blade • #3 handle with 11 blade	• Bonney • smooth • single-tooth Adson • Adson	• Senns	• 10 cc syringe • 2 towel clips • Verres needle • laparoscopic trocar and sleeve (2 10 mm and 1 5 mm) • laparoscope • probe • anti-fog • laparoscopic grasper	1. Prepare a separate basin with Auvard weighted vaginal speculum, Hulka tenaculum, catheter, and open-end speculum. 2. Trocar sizes may vary according to surgeon's preference. 3. Always have open Setup available.

Laparoscopic-Assisted Vaginal Hysterectomy Setup

Core: OB/GYN	Level III

Basic Vaginal Hysterectomy Mayo Setup

Laparoscopy portion will be set up on a Mayo tray with the following:

Scissors	Knives/Scalpels	Forceps	Retractors	Miscellaneous
• laparoscopic	• #3 handle with 10 blade	• single-tooth Adson	• fan	• 10 mm trocar • 5 mm trocar • 5 mm and 10 mm scope • laparoscopic grasper • probe • ligature clips

Back Table Setup (for the vaginal part of the procedure)

Clamps	Knives/Scalpels	Scissors	Forceps	Retractors
• 2 Lahey • 2 curved Heaney • 2 Vanderbilt or Crile • 1 Allis • empty sponge forceps • 1 sponge forceps with	• #3 long handle with 15 blade • #3 handle with 10 blade	• Metzenbaum • curved and straight Mayo • Jorgenson	• Bonney • long multi-tooth Brown • long smooth	• Hasson "S" • Deaver • duckbill vaginal speculum

Myomectomy (Abdominal Approach) Setup

Core: OB/GYN	Level II

Clamps	Knives/Scalpels	Scissors	Forceps	Retractors	Miscellaneous
• 4 cured hemostats • 4 Allis • 4 Kelly • 2 straight Ochsner • 2 sponge sticks loaded with 4 × 4 sponges • towel clip	• #3 handle with 10 blade	• curved Mayo • Metzenbaum • straight Mayo	• Bonney • smooth • Brown multi-tooth	• O'Sullivan-O'Connor	• tenaculum • ESU

Suction Curettage Setup

Core: OB/GYN	Level I

Clamps	Scissors	Forceps	Retractors	Miscellaneous
• 4 sponge forceps	• Mayo • Metzenbaum	• Russian	• Auvard weighted vaginal speculum	• Heaney dilators • tenaculum • curettes • suction cannulas • K-Y jelly

Tubal Ligation Setup

Core: OB/GYN	Level I

Clamps	Knives/Scalpels	Scissors	Forceps	Retractors
• 2 curved hemostat • 2 right angle • 2 Babcock • empty sponge forceps	• 2 #3 handle with 15 blade	• Metzenbaum • straight Mayo	• single-tooth Adson	• Army–Navy

Tuboplasty of Fallopian Tubes Setup

Core: OB/GYN	Level II

Clamps	Knives/Scalpels	Scissors	Forceps	Retractors	Miscellaneous
• 2 curved hemostats • 2 right angle • 2 Babcock • 2 sponge forceps	• #3 handle with 15 blade • #3 handle with 11 blade	• Metzenbaum • straight and curved Mayo • Iris	• Castrovejo suturing with tying platforms • jewelers • single-tooth Adson • DeBakey • Cushing	• 2 Gelpi • 2 small Richardson	• Bowman lacrimal duct probes • bipolar cautery • tongue blade • 18 gauge angiocatheter • syringe with Indigo carmine • may need microscope and microscopic instrumentation

Vaginal Delivery Setup

Core: OB/GYN	Level I

Clamps	Knives/Scalpels	Scissors	Forceps	Miscellaneous
• 2 Ochsner • 2 sponge forceps	• #4 handle with 20 blade • #3 handle with 15 blade	• Metzenbaum • straight and curved Mayo • bandage	• Bonney	• cord clamp • 2 cord blood tubes • bulb syringe • delivery forceps

Vaginal Hysterectomy Setup

Core: OB/GYN	Level II

Clamps	Knives/Scalpels	Scissors	Forceps	Retractors	Miscellaneous	Notes
• 4 curved hemostat • 2 Allis • 4 curved Heaney • 2 straight Heaney • 2 Lahey • 2 sponge forceps with 4 × 4 sponges • 2 Kelly • 4 straight Ochsner • 2 Babcock	• #3 handle with 10 blade • #3 handle with 15 blade	• Metzenbaum • curved and straight Mayo • Jorgenson	• multi-tooth forceps • Bonney • Ferris–Smith • Russian	• Auvard weighted vaginal speculum with glove stretched over the end • 2 Sims • 2 medium Deaver	• tenaculum • basin with red rubber catheter	1. Commonly set up on back table instead of Mayo stand.

Vaginal Sling Setup

Core: OB/GYN	Level I

Clamps	Knives/Scalpels	Scissors	Forceps	Retractors	Notes
• 2 curved hemostats • 2 Crile • 2 Peon or Kelly	• #3 handle with 15 blade	• straight Mayo	• Ferris-Smith	• weighted speculum	1. Cystoscopy may be performed in conjunction with this procedure. This can be set up on a small back table to access as needed: • 2 Kelly • #3 handle with 15 blade • straight Mayo scissors • Adson forceps • DeBakey forceps • Cysto setup: 30 and 70 degree scopes, 18 Foley catheter, 10 cc syringe, sling needle, camera, camera cord, light source, drainage bag, lubricant.

Vulvectomy (Simple) Setup

Specialty: OB/GYN	Level I

Clamps	Knives/Scalpels	Scissors	Forceps	Miscellaneous	Notes
• 4 curved hemostats • 4 Allis	• #3 handle with 10 or 15 blade	• Metzenbaum • curved Mayo • straight Mayo	• Adson multi-tooth • regular smooth	• marking pen • May inject with epinephrine (should be labeled)	1. Lithotomy position usually used. 2. Wound may be left open to granulate. 3. May also do a STSG procedure. 4. Have myocutaneous graft set up in room. 5. Have drain and firm dressing available.

Personal Notes

Personal Notes

Chapter 4

Genitourinary (GU) Surgery

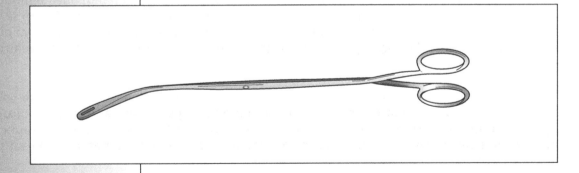

Introduction

Genitourinary surgeries include procedures on both male and female patients. This specialty involves the urinary system, including the kidneys, bladder, urethra, and ureters. It also includes procedures involving the male reproductive system. Urology procedures are classified as either open or closed procedures. An *open procedure* requires an incision, whereas a *closed procedure* is performed through the use of scopes.

Closed procedures

Closed procedures are usually performed in a specialized room called a *cysto room.* During these procedures, the scrub person sets up and works from a back table. In many cases the surgeon and scrub personnel do not have to employ sterile techniques during the procedures. It is important for the surgical team to make sure that they are using the proper irrigating fluid and that it is replaced as needed. The surgical team should remain in the room at all times and have the necessary supplies and proper sizes and equipment.

Considerations during closed procedures may include:

- It is important to use proper topical anesthetic and nonconductive lubricant.
- X-rays are often taken for proper catheter placement; the surgical team needs to use protective equipment.

Open procedures

Open procedures are performed in regular operating rooms. Considerations may include the usage of specialty instruments as well as basic general surgery trays, vascular trays, prostate retractors, and thoracic instrumentation. You may use pedicle clamps and stone forceps. Many varieties of catheters, stents, and guides also must be available.

Considerations following open kidney procedures may include:

- Insertion of chest tubes if the pleural cavity has been entered

List of Procedures

Figure 4-1: Instruments used in a male cystoscopy

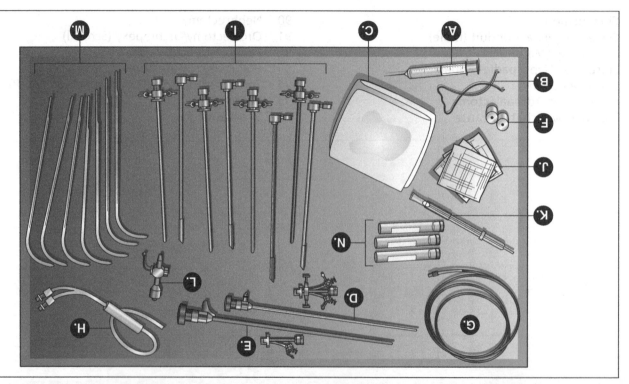

Delmar Cengage Learning

A	local anesthetic loaded into syringe	I	17 French to 25 French obturator and sheath
B	meatus clamp (male)	J	3 × 3 sponges
C	lubricant on towel	K	culture tube
D	30 degree scope with double bridge	L	stopcock
E	70 degree scope with single bridge	M	urethral sounds
F	stoppers	N	test tubes
G	fiberoptic light cord		
H	inflow tubing with stopcock		

Key to Accompany Figure 4-1: Instruments used in a male cystoscopy

Circumcision Setup

Core: GU	Level I

Clamps	Knives/Scalpels	Scissors	Forceps	Miscellaneous	Notes
• 2 small curved hemostat • 4 small straight hemostat • 2 small Allis	• 2 #3 handle with 15 blade	• small Metzenbaum • small straight Mayo	• Adson–Brown • mini-teeth • smooth	• needle point cautery	1. If this procedure is being performed on an infant/toddler, the instrumentation may be smaller or pediatric. 2. Never inject local anesthetic with epinephrine into the penis.

Cystectomy/Ileal Conduit (Male) Setup

Core: GU	Level III

Clamps	Knives/Scalpels	Scissors	Forceps	Retractors	Miscellaneous	Notes
• 4 curved hemostat • 2 straight hemostat • 2 Kelly • 2 Vanderbilt or Criles • 2 right angle (1 short and 1 long) • 1 short and 1 long Babcock • 2 straight Ochsners • 1 curved Ochsner with dissector • 1 sponge forcep with 4 × 4 sponges • 2 non-crushing bowel clamps	• #3 handle with 10 blade • #3 handle with 15 blade • #3 long handle with 10 blade	• Metzenbaum • curved and straight Mayo • long Metzenbaum	• short and long Brown multi-tooth • long DeBakey	• 2 small and 1 medium Richardson	• medium hemoclips • cautery extension **Second Mayo tray setup:** • a large self-retaining abdominal retractor • 2 ribbon retractors	1. Have available in room: stoma bag, Foley catheter with 30 balloon, stapling cart, ureteral stents. 2. In addition to this setup, for a female patient you would need to add instrumentation for a hysterectomy.

Cystoscopy (Male) Back Table Setup

Core: GU	Level I

	Notes
• local anesthetic loaded into syringe • meatus clamp (male) • water-soluble lubricant on towel • 30 degree scope with double bridge • 70 degree scope with single bridge • stoppers • fiberoptic light cord • inflow tubing with stopcock • 17 French to 25 French obturator and sheath • 3 × 3 sponges • culture tubes • stopcock • urethral sounds • test tubes	1. May need catheter and drainage bag to use after the case. 2. For a female you would use cotton swabs with local anesthetic instead of a syringe.

Epispadias/Hypospadias Repair Setup

Core: GU	Level II

Clamps	Knives/Scalpels	Scissors	Forceps	Retractors	Miscellaneous	Notes
• 2 small curved hemostat • 2 small straight hemostat • 1 Allis • curved Ochsner with dissector	• 2 #3 handle with 15 blade	• small Metzenbaum • small straight Metzenbaum • tenotomy	• multi-tooth Adson • smooth	• 2 skin hook	• infant feeding tubes • needle tip cautery • syringe • aspirating needle • probes • pediatric urethral dilators	1. May need catheter.

Hydrocelectomy Setup

Core: GU	Level I

Clamps	Knives/Scalpels	Scissors	Forceps	Retractors	Miscellaneous
• 2 curved hemostat • 2 right angle • 2 Allis • 1 curved Ochsner with dissector	• #3 handle with 10 blade • #3 handle with 15 blade	• small Metzenbaum • straight Metzenbaum	• multi-tooth Adson • regular multi-tooth	• 2 Senn • 2 Army–Navy	• 30 cc syringe with 20 gauge, 2 inch aspirating needle • local anesthetic loaded into syringe with injection needle • Penrose drain

Laparoscopic Adrenalectomy Setup

Core: GU	Level III

Clamps	Knives/Scalpels	Scissors	Forceps	Retractors	Miscellaneous
• 2 Crile • 2 Allis • 2 towel clamps • 1 Kelly • endo grasper • endo right angle	• #3 handle with 11 blade	• neuro Metzenbaums • straight Mayo • endo	• DeBakey • Adsons • endo DeBakey	• S • endo	• endo catch • endo clips • camera and cord • light source • insufflator needle and tubing • endo cautery

Marshall–Marchetti–Krantz Setup

Core: GU	Level I

Clamps	Knives/Scalpels	Scissors	Forceps	Retractors	Miscellaneous
• 4 curved hemostat • 2 straight hemostat • 2 Kelly • 2 Vanderbilt or Crile • 2 right angle • 2 straight Ochsner • 1 curved Ochsner with dissector • 1 sponge forceps with 4 × 4 sponges	• #3 handle with 10 blade • #3 handle with 15 blade • #3 long handle with 10 blade	• Metzenbaum • straight and curved Mayo	• short multi-tooth • 2 pair DeBakey • Bonney	• 2 small Richardson • 1 medium Richardson	• cautery extension • Heaney needle holders

Nephrectomy Setup

Core: GU	Level III

Clamps	Knives/Scalpels	Scissors	Forceps	Retractors	Miscellaneous	Notes
• 4 curved hemostat • 2 straight hemostat • 2 Kelly • 2 Vanderbilt or Crile • 2 long right angle • 2 short right angle • 2 straight Ochsner • 2 curved Ochsner loaded with dissector • 2 curved sponge forceps with 4 × 4 sponges • Mayo pedicle clamp • vascular clamps	• #4 handle with 20 blade • #3 handle with 10 blade • #3 long handle with 10 blade	• long Metzenbaum • long straight Metzenbaum • curved and straight Mayo • Potts–Smith	• long multi-tooth • 2 pair long DeBakey • Bonney • regular multi-tooth	• 2 small Richardson • 2 vein	• right angle hemoclips • medium and large hemoclips • Alexander • Doyen • rib shears • rib rongeurs • cautery extension **Second Mayo Tray Setup:** Retractors: 3 Deaver, 2 heart-shaped, 2 ribbon, and a large self-retaining retractor	1. May need chest tubes and drainage system at the end of the procedure.

Orchiectomy/Orchiopexy (Scrotal) Setup

Core: GU	Level I

Clamps	Knives/Scalpels	Scissors	Forceps	Retractors	Miscellaneous
• 2 curved hemostat • 2 straight hemostat • 2 Allis	• 2 #3 handle with 15 blade	• small curved Metzenbaum • straight Metzenbaum	• multi-tooth Adson • smooth	• 2 Senn • 2 skin hook	• needle tip Cautery

Penile Implant Setup

Core: GU	Level II

Clamps	Knives/Scalpels	Scissors	Forceps	Retractors	Miscellaneous	Notes
• 2 curved hemostat • 2 straight hemostat • 2 Allis	• 2 #3 handle with 15 blade	• small Metzenbaum • regular Metzenbaum • straight Mayo	• multi-tooth Adson • regular multi-tooth • regular smooth	• 2 Senn • 2 Army–Navy	• Hegar dilators • inserter • closing tool • clamping connectors • Foley catheter • Keith needles • local anesthetic • methylene blue • ruler • Andrews suction tip	1. Have the surgeon's preference of penile prosthesis available.

(Radical) Prostatectomy Setup

Core: GU		Level III	

Clamps	Knives/Scalpels	Scissors	Forceps	Retractors	Miscellaneous	Notes
• 4 curved hemostat • 2 straight hemostat • 2 Kelly • 2 Vanderbilt • 2 long right angle • 2 long Allis • 2 straight Ochsner • 1 curved Ochsner • 2 curved Ochsner with dissector • 1 right McDougle • 2 curved sponge forceps with 4 × 4 sponges	• #4 handle with 20 blade • #3 handle with 10 blade • #3 long handle with 15 blade	• long curved and straight Metzenbaum • regular Metzenbaum • curved and straight Mayo	• long multi-tooth • long smooth • long DeBakey • Bonney • regular multi-tooth • long Russian • 2 pair delicate single-tooth	• 2 small Richardson • 2 vein • 2 Army–Navy	• large and medium hemoclips • right angle • clips • cautery extension • Heaney needle holders • Van Buren urethral sounds • lubricant	1. Have Deaver retractors and large self-retaining retractor ready on back table.

Transurethral Resection of Prostate (TURP) Back Table Setup

Core: GU	Level I

- water-soluble lubricant
- Van Buren dilators
- sheaths
- obturators
- resectoscope with working element
- inflow tubing
- light cord
- catheter guide
- Ellik evacuator
- Toomey syringe
- cautery cord
- 22 French 3-way 30 cc Foley and drainage bag (or size of surgeon's preference)
- cutting loops
- telescope
- rubber tips
- stopcock
- syringe

Vasectomy Setup

Core: GU	Level I

Clamps	Knives/Scalpels	Scissors	Forceps	Retractors	Miscellaneous
• 2 curved mosquito • 2 small Allis	• #3 handle with 15 blade	• small curved and straight Metzenbaum	• multi-tooth Adson	• 2 Senn • 2 Joseph skin hook	• 10 cc syringe and 27 gauge needle • local anesthetic • needle tip cautery • 2 towel clips

Vasovasostomy Setup

Core: GU	Level II

Clamps	Knives/Scalpels	Scissors	Forceps	Retractors	Miscellaneous	Notes
• 2 small curved hemostat • 2 small straight hemostat • 1 Babcock	• 2 #3 handle with 15 blade	• small curved and straight Metzenbaum	• multi-tooth Adson • smooth	• 2 Senn • 2 skin hook	• glass slide • Bowman tear duct probe or dilators • approximator clip	1. If using a microscope you will need to add: • 2 microscopic curved smooth forceps • 1 microscopic tissue forceps • 1 microscopic curved tying forceps • Castroviejo needle holder • Vas holder

Personal Notes

Personal Notes

Personal Notes

Personal Notes

Personal Notes

Chapter 5

Thoracic Surgery

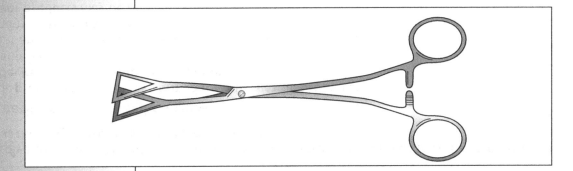

Introduction

Thoracic procedures involve surgical intervention on the chest and thoracic cavity and organs that are included within this region, such as the lungs, bronchus, and the mediastinum.

Considerations for thoracic procedures might include:

- Endoscopic diagnostic procedures may be performed prior to surgical procedure.
- Various positioning devices may be used for best exposure.
- Procedures may be lengthy.
- Specialized equipment and supplies, such as stapling instrumentation, may be used.
- Chest tube and drainage systems may be used.
- Blood and replacement products may be needed.
- Special anesthesia equipment must be available.

List of Procedures

Bronchoscopy Setup

- suction
- 25 gauge needle
- Telfa
- biopsy forceps
- bronchoscope
- light cord
- anesthetic spray
- Lukens specimen trap
- endotracheal adapter
- small basin with sterile saline
- lubricant
- bronchoscopy brush
- syringe
- straight Mayo scissors
- test tube

Mediastinoscopy Setup

Specialty: Cardiothoracic	Level II

Clamps	Knives/Scalpels	Scissors	Forceps	Retractors	Miscellaneous	Notes
• 3 curved hemostat • 1 straight hemostat • 2 right angle • 1 curved Ochsner loaded with dissector	• #3 handle with 15 blade	• Metzenbaum • curved and straight Mayo	• smooth • Brown multi-tooth • DeBakey	• 2 Senn • 2 Army–Navy • 2 small Richardson • 1 medium Gelpi	• mediastino-scope • fiberoptic light source • scope suction • biopsy forceps • needle and as-piration tube • Staimey needle • Luer-lock syringe • Frazier suction • mediastinos-copy suction tip	1. The position of the Mayo tray varies according to the position of the anesthesia personnel and equipment, and access to the operative site by the surgeon.

Pacemaker Insertion Setup

Specialty: Cardiothoracic	Level II

Clamps	Knives/Scalpels	Scissors	Forceps	Retractors	Miscellaneous
• 2 curved mosquito • 4 curved hemostat • 2 right angle • 2 DeBakey vascular clamps	• #3 handle with 15 blade • #3 handle with 11 blade	• Metzenbaum • straight Mayo • Potts–Smith	• DeBakey • smooth • Brown multi-tooth	• 2 small Richardson • 2 small Weitlaner • 2 Senn • 2 blunt rake	• tunneler • hemoclips • syringe loaded with local anesthetic and injection needle of surgeon's preference • pacemaker generator • electrodes • alligator clips • vessel loops • Frazier suction tip

Scalene Node Biopsy Setup

Specialty: Cardiothoracic | **Level I**

Clamps	Knives/Scalpels	Scissors	Forceps	Retractors
• 4 curved hemostat • 1 Kelly • 2 right angle • 2 Allis • 2 curved Ochsner with dissectors	• 2 #3 handle with 15 blade	• straight and curved Mayo • Metzenbaum	• Brown multi-tooth • DeBakey	• 2 small Richardson • 2 Senn • 2 Weitlaner

Thoracoscopy Setup

Specialty: Cardiothoracic | **Level II**

Miscellaneous	Endoscopic	Notes
• camera • light cord • 10 mm 0 and 30 degree lens • 2 curved hemostat clamps • 2 small Richardson retractors • 2 #3 handle with 15 blade • straight Mayo scissors • 1 Kelly clamp • anti-fog • 2 10 mm trocars • 12 mm trocar • reducers • irrigating tubing • local anesthetic and syringe/needle of surgeon's preference	• blunt grasper • serrated grasper • cautery cord • suture carrier • Pennington forceps • lung retractor • hemoclips • hooked scissors • micro scissors • straight scissors • probe • dissector	1. Have major set and vascular set of instruments available in room. 2. Chest tubes and drainage system will be used following the procedure.

Thoracotomy Setup

Specialty: Cardiothoracic | Level II

Clamps	Knives/Scalpels	Scissors	Forceps	Retractors	Miscellaneous	Notes
• 4 curved hemostat • 2 straight hemostat • 2 Kelly • 2 Vanderbilt or Criles • 2 right angle • 2 Mixter • vascular clamps • 2 curved Ochsner with dissectors • 2 sponge forceps with 4 × 4 sponges • 3 straight Ochsner	• #4 handle with 20 blade • #3 handle with 10 blade • #3 long handle with 15 blade	• long and regular Metzenbaum • curved and straight Mayo	• 3 Duval lung • Brown multi-tooth (regular and long) • smooth • 2 pair DeBakey • Russian	• self-retaining chest retractor • 2 small Richardson • 1 medium Richardson • 2 Harrington	• 2 Doyen elevators • Alexander periostotome • rib approximator	1. A separate Mayo may be used for holding the retractors instead of placing them on the primary Mayo tray. 2. Chest tubes and drainage system will be used following the procedure. 3. Special positioning devices may be used. 4. Have a set of extra-long instruments available. 5. This Mayo setup may be used for: pneumonectomy, decortication, lobectomy, lung biopsy.

Personal Notes

Chapter 6

Cardiovascular (CV) Surgery

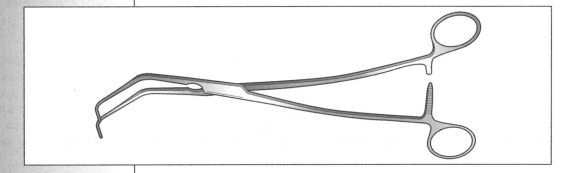

Introduction

Cardiovascular procedures include those performed on the heart and the great vessels that are associated with the circulatory system, such as the aorta and the coronary arteries. This specialty is separated from the thoracic and peripheral vascular system because of the complexity of the procedures that are performed on the heart and great vessels. Details and anticipation are a necessity when doing cardiovascular procedures. Because you are working with veins and arteries, you will be using various suture materials, vessel loops, umbilical tapes, and suture boots. Some people choose to have these on their Mayo setup for easy access.

AST Specialty: Cardiothoracic

Considerations for cardiovascular procedures include:

- Specialty instrumentation and large setups
- Multiple Mayo setups, which may include a Mayo setup for cannulation
- Limited exposure
- Bypass grafting and vein harvesting
- Chest closure
- Extracorporeal (heart–lung bypass machine) circulation supplies
- Pacemakers
- Chest tubes and drainage systems
- Cooling equipment
- Lengthy procedures
- Delicate instrumentation and suturing equipment
- Be prepared for urgent situations
- Specialty suture used in large amounts

List of Procedures

Aortic Valve Replacement Setup

Specialty: Cardiothoracic	Level III

	Notes
Coronary Artery Bypass Setup (see page 125) with the addition of the following instruments: • 4 Allis clamps • suture ring • valve holder • 2 medium Richardson retractors • valve retractor • valve dilators or obturator • aortic valve sizers • aortic valve dilators • dental mirror • valve hook • valve scissors • rongeur	1. Keep track of the many suture needles used on the field. 2. Attention to detail is critical. 3. Be prepared for emergent situations. 4. Prosthesis should not be opened until surgeon requests needed size. 5. Keep instrument tips clean with moistened sponge.

Coronary Artery Bypass Setup

Specialty: Cardiothoracic	Level III

Clamps	Knives/Scalpels	Scissors	Forceps	Miscellaneous	Notes
• 2 mosquito • 2 mosquito hemostat clamps loaded with suture boots • 4 curved hemostat • 4 Crile • 4 right angle • 6 tubing clamps • 4 Kelly • partial occlusion clamp • 2 Craford • 2 DeBakey • 2 Satinsky • 2 Cooley • 2 straight vascular clamps	• 2 #10 handle with 3 blade • #7 handle with 15 blade • #7 handle with 11 blade • #64 Beaver blade and handle • #4 handle with 20 blade	• Metzenbaum • straight Mayo • Potts–Smith • Jameson • coronary scissors: right angle, angled, backbiter	• 2 pair Brown multi-tooth • 2 pair DeBakey • 1 pair Russian • Potts–Smith tissue **Retractors** • sternum self-retaining • 2 small Richardson • 1 medium Richardson • 2 vein	• coronary dilators • marking pen • bulldog clamps • aortic punch • ruler • aortic dilator • hemoclips: small, medium, large, and right angle • coronary Freer elevator • Rumel tourniquet • heparin irrigation loaded into syringe • sump catheter • pace maker wires • bone wax	1. Because of the excessive supplies needed for this procedure, some people use a Mayfield table in addition to the Mayo tray to have their instruments accessible. Also, some supplies are left on the back table until ready for use, such as the sternal wiring supplies. 2. The following supplies will also be needed and may have special places within your sterile field instead of being on the already crowded Mayo tray: • bypass tubing • sternal saw • internal defibrillator paddles • slush • internal mammary retractor • chest wires loaded on Ochsner clamps • wire twisters • wire cutters • closed-seal drainage • vein retrieval instruments

Mitral Valve Replacement Setup

Specialty: Cardiothoracic	Level III

	Notes
Coronary Artery Bypass Setup with the addition of the following instruments. • 4 Allis clamps • suture ring • valve holder • 2 medium Richardson retractors • valve retractor • valve dilators or obturator • mitral valve sizers • dental mirror • valve hook • valve scissors • rongeur	1. Keep track of the many suture needles used on the field. 2. Attention to detail is critical. 3. Be prepared for emergent situations. 4. Prosthesis should not be opened until surgeon requests needed size. 5. Keep instrument tips clean with moistened sponge.

Pericardial Window Setup

Specialty: Cardiothoracic | **Level II**

Clamps	Knives/Scalpels	Scissors	Forceps	Retractors	Miscellaneous	Notes
• 4 curved hemostat • 2 right angle • 2 Allis • 1 Kelly • 2 Vanderbilt or Crile • 2 curved Ochsner with dissectors	• #3 handle with 10 blade • #3 handle with 15 blade	• Metzenbaum • Jameson • straight and curved Mayo	• Brown multi-tooth • 2 pair DeBakey	• 2 small Richardson • 1 medium Richardson • sternal	• sternal saw • chest tube passer • bone wax • 6 sternal wires loaded on Ochsner clamps • wire twister • wire driver • wire cutter	1. Have prolene suture loaded with pledgets. 2. Have bypass supplies ready.

Sternum Rewiring Setup

Specialty: Cardiothoracic	Level I

Clamps	Knives/Scalpels	Scissors	Forceps	Retractors	Miscellaneous
• 2 curved hemostat • 2 Kelly • 10 straight Ochsner	• #3 handle with 10 blade • #3 handle with 15 blade	• Metzenbaum • curved and straight Mayo	• 2 pair Brown multi-tooth	• 2 small Richardson	• rongeurs • wire twister • wire cutters • wire driver • bone wax

Thoracic Aortic Aneurysm Repair Setup

Specialty: Cardiothoracic	Level III

Abdominal Aortic Aneurysm
Repair setup with the following
additions:
- rib spreader
- Doyen coastal elevator
- periosteal elevator
- chest tube passer
- lung clamp
- chest retractor

Thymectomy Setup

Specialty: Cardiothoracic | **Level II**

Clamps	Knives/Scalpels	Scissors	Forceps	Retractors	Miscellaneous
• 4 curved hemostat • 2 straight hemostat • 2 Kelly • 4 Schnidt hemostat • 4 right angle • 4 Allis • 4 straight Ochsner • 2 curved Ochsner with dissector sponges • 2 sponge forceps with 4 × 4 sponges • 2 angled vascular clamp • 4 straight vascular clamp	• #4 handle with 20 blade • #3 handle with 10 blade • #3 long handle with 15 blade	• curved Mayo • straight Mayo • regular and long Metzenbaum	• regular and long Brown multi-tooth • long smooth • regular and long DeBakey • Ferris-Smith	• sternum • 2 small Richardson • medium Richardson • large rake	• bovie extension • hemoclips • power sternal saw • bone wax • chest wires • wire cutter • wire twister • wire driver

Vein Retrieval Setup

Specialty: Cardiothoracic	Level I

Clamps	Knives/Scalpels	Scissors	Forceps	Retractors	Miscellaneous
• 2 curved mosquito • 2 curved hemostat • 2 small right angle • 2 medium right angle • 1 Kelly	• #3 handle with 15 blade • #3 handle with 11 blade	• Potts–Smith • Jameson • Metzenbaum • straight Mayo	• 2 pair DeBakey • Brown multi-tooth	• 2 Senn • 2 small Richardson • 1 vein • 2 Army–Navy • 2 Weitlaner	• heparin irrigation loaded into syringe with blunt needle • hemoclips • vessel cannula

Personal Notes

Personal Notes

Chapter 7

Peripheral Vascular (PV) Surgery

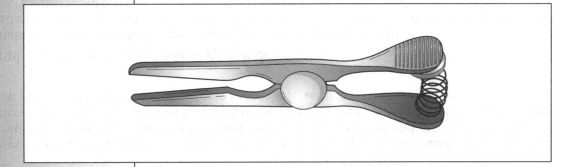

Introduction

This specialty involves procedures performed on the portion of the circulatory system that supplies blood to the brain, organs, and extremities. These arteries and veins ultimately interact with the heart and great vessels to supply necessary blood to all parts of the body. The surgeries involving the arteries and veins within the peripheral vascular specialty also require great detail and knowledge to facilitate proper intervention so that procedures can be carried out successfully.

Considerations for peripheral vascular procedures may include:

- Various suture materials, vessel loops, umbilical tapes, and suture boots will be needed.
- Multiple drugs, irrigation solutions, and other solutions will be on the field. Every precaution necessary to avoid confusing drugs should be taken. All medications should be labeled.
- All syringes and basins/containers should be labeled.
- Various types and sizes of grafts and patch material should be available in the room.

List of Procedures

Abdominal Aortic Aneurysm Repair Setup

Specialty: Peripheral Vascular	Level III

Clamps	Knives/Scalpels	Scissors	Forceps	Retractors	Miscellaneous	Notes
• 4 curved mosquito hemostat (2 loaded with suture boots) • 4 curved hemostat • 2 straight hemostat • 2 Kelly • 4 Vanderbilt or Crile • 4 right angle • 2 Allis • 3 straight Ochsner • 2 sponge forceps loaded with 4 × 4 sponges • 2 curved Ochsner loaded with dissectors • 2 DeBakey curved vascular • 2 straight vascular • 1 aortic clamp • 2 angled DeBakey vascular • 2 curved Craford vascular	• #4 handle with 20 blade • #3 handle with 10 blade • #3 long handle with 15 blade	• regular and long Metzenbaum • curved and straight Mayo	• 2 pair DeBakey • regular and long Brown multi-tooth • 2 pair Russian • long smooth	• 2 small Richardson	• Rumel tourniquet • Freer elevator • hemoclips **Second Mayo Tray Setup:** Retractors: • 2 medium and 1 large Richardson • 1 narrow, 1 medium, and 1 wide Deaver • 2 Harrington • 2 ribbon • extra-wide Deaver • Balfour • large self-retaining retractor	1. Pre-clotting of graft may be required. 2. Have a variety of grafts available. 3. May use large self-retaining retractor such as Bookwalter or Thompson.

Aortic Bi-femoral Bypass Setup

Specialty: Peripheral Vascular	Level III

The Mayo tray setup will be the same as for an Abdominal Aortic Aneurysm Repair, with the following additions:

Clamps	Forceps	Retractors	Miscellaneous	Notes
• 4 curved hemostat • 2 regular right angle • 4 short-angled vascular • 4 curved vascular • Statinsky • 2 Kelly • 2 short right angle • 2 curved Ochsner loaded with dissectors • 4 Criles or Vanderbilts	• 2 pair regular DeBakey • Brown multi-tooth	• 4 Weitlaner • 2 small Richardson	• tunneler	1. Have bifurcated grafts available in various sizes. 2. Will need heparinized saline for flushing. 3. Many need sterile doppler probe. 4. May do arteriogram.

Arteriovenous Fistula Setup

Specialty: Peripheral Vascular	Level II

Mayo setup or back table setup

Clamps	Knives/Scalpels	Scissors	Forceps	Retractors	Miscellaneous	Notes
• 2 mosquito hemostat • 2 curved hemostat • 1 Kelly • 2 right angle • 1 Allis • 1 curved Ochsner with dissector • 2 angled vascular • 2 straight vascular • 2 curved vascular	• #3 handle with 15 blade • #3 handle with 11 blade	• Metzen-baum • suture • Potts–Smith • Jameson	• Brown multi-tooth • 2 pair DeBakey	• 2 small Richardson • 2 Senn • 2 Gelpi • 2 Weitlaner	• vessel dilators • Rumel tourniquet • tunneler • bulldog clamps • heparinized saline loaded into a syringe for irrigation with blunt needle or preferred irrigation tip	1. Have vascular grafts available in the room. 2. Mayo setup may also be used for arteriovenous shunt and removal of infected graft. 3. Will need heparinized saline to flush artery. 4. May need sterile doppler probe.

Axillofemoral Bypass Setup

Specialty: Peripheral Vascular | **Level II**

Clamps	Knives/Scalpels	Scissors	Forceps	Retractors	Miscellaneous	Notes
• 2 curved mosquito • 4 curved hemostat • 2 straight hemostat • 2 Kelly • 2 right angle • 2 curved Ochsner with dissector • 2 angled vascular • 2 right angle vascular • 2 straight vascular	• #3 handle with 10 blade • #3 handle with 15 blade • #3 handle with 11 blade	• short and regular Metzenbaum • Jameson • straight Mayo • Potts–Smith	• Brown multi-tooth • 2 pair DeBakey	• 2 small Richardson • 2 Army–Navy • 4 Weitlaner • 1 medium Richardson	• Rumel tourniquet • heparinized saline in syringe • tunneler • vessel loops • umbilical tapes	1. Have grafts available in the room; also have vascular patch material available. 2. Heparinized saline will be used for flushing. 3. May need sterile doppler probe. 4. May do arteriogram.

Carotid Endarterectomy Setup

Specialty: Peripheral Vascular | **Level II**

Clamps	Knives/Scalpels	Scissors	Forceps	Retractors	Miscellaneous	Notes
• 2 curved mosquito • 4 curved hemostat • 3 straight hemostat • 2 right angle • 2 curved Ochsner with dissectors • 2 angled vascular • 1 Satinsky vascular • 2 curved vascular	• 2 #3 handle with 15 blade • #3 handle with 11 blade	• Jameson • tenotomy • Potts–Smith • regular and short Metzenbaum • suture	• Brown multi-tooth • Russian • 2 pair DeBakey	• 2 Weitlaner • 2 small Richardson	• shunt clamps • heparinized irrigation • 2 Freer elevators	1. Have shunts available according to surgeon's preference. 2. Have graft patch material available. 3. Have heparinized saline available for flushing. 4. May need sterile doppler probe. 5. May need 1% lidocaine or papaverine on field. 6. Label all medications.

Embolectomy Setup

Specialty: Peripheral Vascular	Level II

Clamps	Knives/Scalpels	Scissors	Forceps	Retractors	Miscellaneous	Notes
• 4 curved hemostat • 2 mosquito hemostat • 2 right angle • 2 striaght and 2 curved vascular (these may vary according to surgeon's preference)	• #3 handle with 15 blade • #3 handle with 11 blade	• Metzenbaum • tenotomy • Potts • striaght Mayo	• Brown multi-tooth • 2 pair DeBakey • Adson multi-tooth	• 2 Weitlaner or Gelpi • 2 small Richardson	• embolectomy catheter (such as Fogarty) • 3 cc syringe • TB syringe • heparinzed saline and needle for flush • contrast medium loaded into syringe • stopcock • IV tubing	1. Fluoroscopy is often used. 2. May need sterile doppler probe. 3. May need vessel loops. 4. Specimen (thrombus or clots) may be sent to pathology. 5. Label all medications on field.

Femoral–Popliteal Bypass Setup

Specialty: Peripheral Vascular	Level II

Clamps	Knives/Scalpels	Scissors	Forceps	Retractors	Miscellaneous	Notes
• 2 curved mosquito • 4 curved hemostat • 1 Kelly • 2 right angle • 2 curved Ochsner with dissectors • 2 bulldog • 2 angled vascular • 2 curved vascular • 2 Satinsky vascular	• #3 handle with 10 blade • #3 handle with 15 blade • #3 handle with 11 blade	• regular and short Metzenbaum • suture • Potts–Smith • Jameson	• regular Brown multi-tooth • 2 pair DeBakey	• 2 small Richardson • 2 Weitlaner • 1 medium Richardson	• tunneler • heparin irrigation • Rumel tourniquet • Freer elevator • hemoclips	1. May need valvulatome and vessel cannula. Also need to have grafts available. 2. Mayo setup may also be used for any femoral–distal bypass or popliteal–distal bypass lower extremity, or femoral-to-femoral bypass. 3. May need sterile doppler probe. 4. May need heparinized saline for flushing. 5. May do an arteriogram.

Vein Ligation Setup

Specialty: Peripheral Vascular	Level I

Clamps	Knives/Scalpels	Scissors	Forceps	Retractors	Notes
• 2 mosquito hemostat • 4 curved hemostat • 1 Kelly • 2 right angle • 1 angled vascular	• #3 handle with 15 blade • #3 handle with 11 blade	• Metzenbaum • curved and straight Mayo • Jameson	• Brown multi-tooth • 2 pair DeBakey	• 2 Weitlaner • 2 small Richardson	1. If doing a vein stripping, add a vein stripper with various tips.

Personal Notes

Personal Notes

Personal Notes

Chapter 8

Orthopedic Surgery

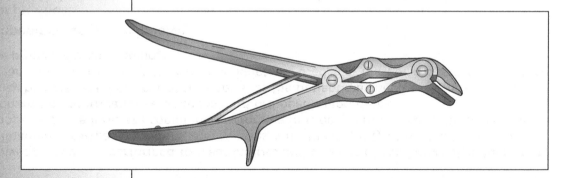

Introduction

Orthopedic surgery involves procedures performed to treat injuries and diseases of the body's skeletal system, including bones, joints, ligaments, cartilage, tendons, and muscles, with the majority of procedures being done on the extremities. Orthopedic procedures are commonly performed in rooms with laminar airflow systems, to reduce the risk of infection. Antibiotic irrigations are used in most orthopedic procedures.

Surgical procedures may be performed on specialized tables, or the patient may need additional positioning devices such as pillows, bean bags, frames, and so forth. If tourniquets are used, they must be properly placed on the limb and the skin must be protected with padding.

Considerations in orthopedic surgery may involve:

- The use of implants or prostheses.
- The use of special implants for joint replacements and various systems for fracture repairs, and the accompanying instrumentation.
- Power instruments must be connected properly.
- Power instruments should never be submerged in water.
- Instrumentation may be heavy and sharp and must be handled properly to protect edges.
- Numerous sets of instruments may be needed for certain procedures.
- Great detail should be given to sterilization techniques to reduce the risk of infection.
- Some surgeons require a 10-minute surgical scrub preparation and require personnel to double-glove during the procedure, and wear hood coverings over hair.

List of Procedures

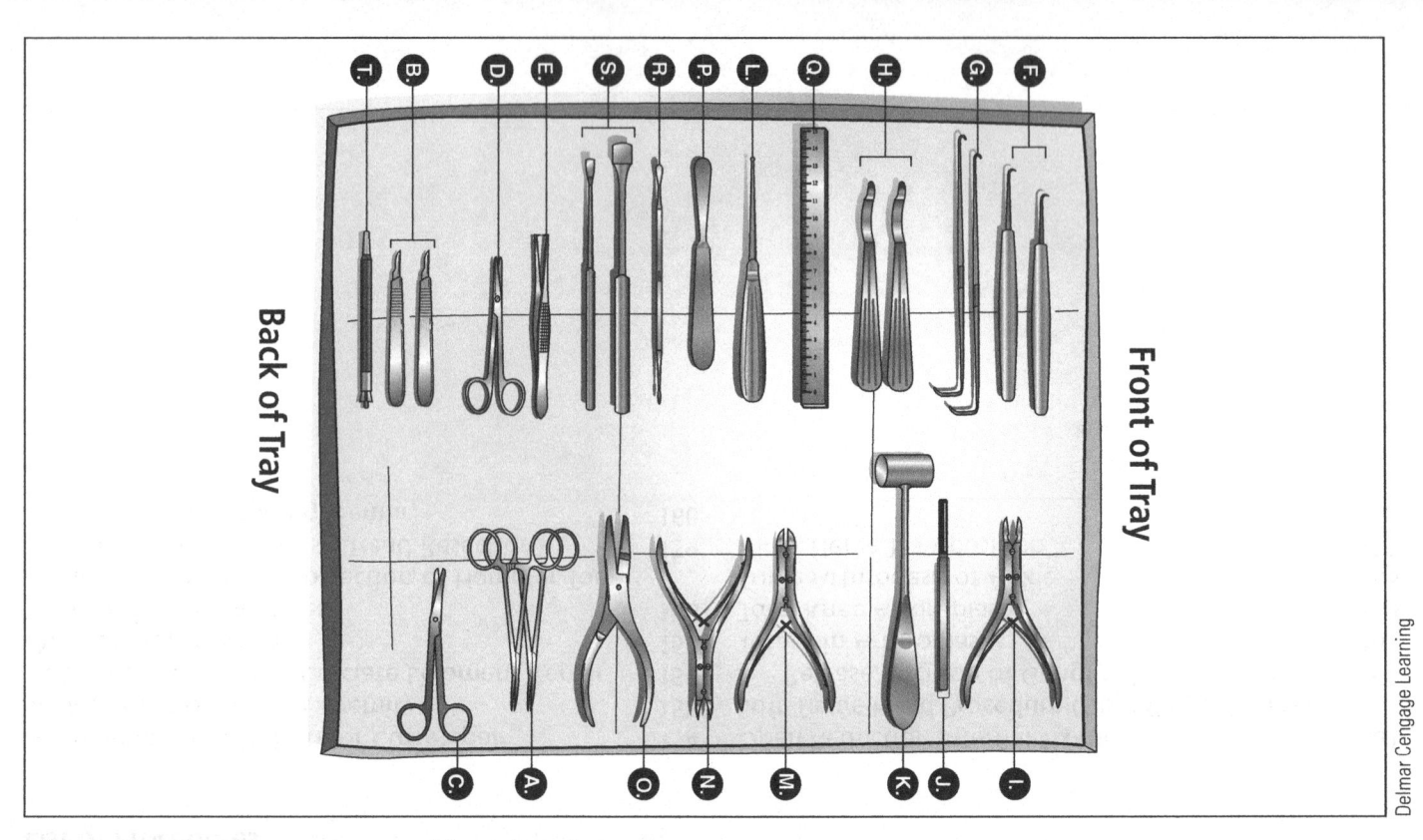

Back of Tray

Front of Tray

Figure 8-1: Instruments used in a bunionectomy

CLAMPS:

A   curved hemostat

KNIVES/SCALPELS:

B   #3 handle with 15 blade

SCISSORS:

C   small Metzenbaum
D   straight Mayo

FORCEPS:

E   single-tooth Adson

RETRACTORS:

F   skin hook
G   Senn
H   small Hohmann

MISCELLANEOUS:

I   small rongeur
J   small osteotome
K   small mallet
L   small cup curette
M   bone cutter
N   pin cutter
O   needle nose pliers
P   rasp
Q   ruler
R   Freer elevator
S   1/4" key elevator
T   marking pen

Key to Accompany Figure 8-1: Instruments used in a bunionectomy

Acromioplasty with Rotator Cuff Repair Setup

Core: Orthopedic	Level I

Clamps	Knives/Scalpels	Scissors	Forceps	Retractors	Miscellaneous	Notes
• 2 curved hemostat • 2 straight hemostat • 2 straight Ochsner	• #3 handle with 10 blade • #3 handle with 15 blade	• small Metzenbaum • regular Metzenbaum • curved Mayo • straight Mayo	• single-tooth Adson • Bonney • regular single-tooth	• Army–Navy • Volkman rake, 2-prong • small Richardson • small Hohmann • Bankart • Gelpi	• small cup curette • small straight osteotome • mallet • small straight rongeur • gooseneck rongeur • small rasp • Freer elevator • 1/4" key elevator • marking pen	1. Have available small oscillating saw, small burrs, power drill, and rotator cuff anchors.

Amputation of Lower Extremity Setup

Core: Orthopedic	Level I

Clamps	Knives/Scalpels	Scissors	Forceps	Retractors	Miscellaneous	Notes
• 2 curved hemostat • 2 straight hemostat • 2 straight Ochsner	• amputation knife • 2 #3 handle with 10 blade • #3 handle with 15 blade • #4 handle with 20 blade	• small Metzenbaum • regular Metzenbaum • curved Mayo • straight Mayo	• single-tooth Adson • Bonney	• Volkman	• bone cutter • rongeurs, small and medium • rasp • 1/2" key elevator • marking pen	1. Have Gigli or power saw available.

Arthroscopic Anterior Cruciate Ligament Repair Setup

Core: Orthopedic	Level III

Same as Knee Arthroscopy with the following additions:

Clamps	Knives/Scalpels	Scissors	Forceps	Retractors	Miscellaneous	Notes
• 2 straight Ochsner • 2 curved hemostat	• #3 handle with 15 blade • extra 15 blades • disposable double-bladed	• small and regular Metzenbaum • curved Mayo	• Bonney	• Senn • small rakes	• marking pen • cautery • small ronguer • small periosteal elevators • curettes • osteotomes • ruler • bone tamp • ACL Guide System • bone tunnel plugs • fixation device • power drill • micro-sag saw • 4.5 arthroscopic bur • arthroscopic osteotome and rasp	1. Make area on back table available for surgeon to work on graft. 2. Save all bone chips.

Arthroscopy of Knee Setup

Core: Orthopedic	Level II

Clamps	Knives/Scalpels	Scissors	Forceps	Miscellaneous	Notes
• straight hemostat	• #3 handle with 15 blade • #3 handle with 11 blade	• suture	• single-tooth Adson	• 60 cc Luer-Lock syringe with 18 gauge needle filled with saline • inflow cannula • blunt trocar and cannula (check surgeon's preference for size) • 30 degree arthroscope (check surgeon's preference for degree of scope) • blunt nerve hook • meniscal biter • meniscal scissors • meniscal grasper • spinal needle • camera • shaving system • inflow/outflow tubing • irrigation system	1. Have local anesthetic and steroid injections available. 2. Have shavers and burrs for shaving system available.

Arthroscopy of Shoulder Setup

| Core: Orthopedic | Level II |

Same as Arthroscopy of Knee setup with additional:

Miscellaneous	Notes
• Shoulder arthroscopy set that would include switching sticks and a Wissinger rod. Variety of fixation devices (screws, staples, or suture). Power drill may be necessary. Cautery may be used.	1. Depending on surgeon's preference, patient may be in lateral or beach-chair position. Traction devices and weights will be used.

Bunionectomy Setup

Core: Orthopedic	Level I

Clamps	Knives/Scalpels	Scissors	Forceps	Retractors	Miscellaneous	Notes
• 2 curved hemostat	• 2 #3 handle with 15 blade	• small Metzenbaum • straight Mayo	• single-tooth Adson	• 2 skin hooks • Senn • 2 small Hohmann	• small rongeur • small osteotome • small mallet • small cup curette • bone cutter • pin cutter • needle nose pliers • rasp • ruler • Freer elevator • 1/4" key elevator • marking pen	1. Have available small sag saw, burrs, power drill, K-wires, any implantables, and small fragment and cannulated screws. 2. Mayo setup may also be used for: correction of hammer toe deformity, metatarsal head resection.

Intramedullary Rodding (Femur) Setup

Core: Orthopedic	Level II

Clamps	Knives/Scalpels	Scissors	Forceps	Retractors	Miscellaneous	Notes
• 2 curved hemostat • 2 straight Ochsner	• #3 handle with 10 blade • #3 handle with 15 blade	• Metzenbaum • curved and straight Mayo	• Brown multi-tooth • single-tooth Adson • Bonney	• 2 Army–Navy • 2 4-prong rake	• 1 medium curette • 1 small elevator • 1 rongeur • pliers • mallet • awl • threaded guide pin • reamer gauge • skin protector • guide rod holder • nail length gauge • medullary exchange tube • hex-head screw driver	1. Have available on the back table: guide rods, wires, cannulated reamers, drill, proximal drill guide, and slap hammer with nail and inserter. 2. If using a locking nail, add the following: drill sleeves, self-tapping locking screws, and targeting device. 3. Have a curved-tip guide pin available.

Open Reduction Internal Fixation Setup

Core: Orthopedic	Level II

This is a generic Mayo setup. The size of instrumentation would change depending on which bone is fractured.

Clamps	Knives/Scalpels	Scissors	Forceps	Retractors	Miscellaneous	Notes
• 2 curved hemostat • 2 straight Ochsner	• 2 #3 handles with 10 blade • #3 handle with 15 blade	• curved Mayo • straight Mayo • Metzenbaum	• single-tooth Adson • Bonney	• Senn • Volkman rake, 2-prong • Hohmann • Bennett • Gelpi	• osteotome • mallet • curettes • rongeur • screwdriver • depth gauge • bone clamps • Freer elevator • key elevators • ruler • marking pen	1. Have appropriate plates and screws available, as well as power drills, K-wires, and lavage system.

Soft-Tissue Hand Procedure Setup

Core: Orthopedic	Level I

Clamps	Knives/Scalpels	Scissors	Forceps	Retractors	Miscellaneous	Notes
• 2 small curved hemostat • 1 small Allis	• 2 #3 handle with 15 blade	• small Metzenbaum • tenotomy • iris • suture	• single-tooth Adson	• skin hooks • Senn • small Gelpi	• Freer elevator • small rongeur • marking pen	1. Have local anesthetic injection available. 2. Mayo setup may also be used for: carpal tunnel release, excision of ganglion.

Total Hip Arthroplasty Setup

Core: Orthopedic	Level III

Clamps	Knives/Scalpels	Scissors	Forceps	Retractors	Miscellaneous	Notes
• 2 curved hemostat • 2 straight Ochsner	• 4 #3 handle with 10 blade • #3 long handle with 15 blade • #4 handle with 20 blade	• curved Mayo • straight Mayo • Metzenbaum	• Ferris–Smith • Bonney	• large Gelpi • large rake • 2 Hohmann • Bennett • Meyerding • Charnley	• 1/2" osteotome and 1" straight osteotome • straight rongeur • gooseneck rongeur • medium cup curette • small long curette • mallet • 1/2" key elevator • medium Cobb elevator • bone hook • nerve hook • box cutter • T-reamer • pliers • marking pen	1. Have reciprocating saw, acetabular reamers, and lavage available. 2. Have implant system available.

Total Knee Arthroplasty Setup

Core: Orthopedic	Level III

Clamps	Knives/Scalpels	Scissors	Forceps	Retractors	Miscellaneous	Notes
• 2 towel clips • 2 curved hemostat • 2 straight Ochsner	• 4 #3 handle with 10 blade • #3 handle with 15 blade • #4 handle with 20 blade	• curved Mayo • straight Mayo • Metzenbaum	• Bonney • single-tooth	• large Gelpi • Volkman rake, 2-prong • Z-retractor (Doane knee retractor) • Hohmann	• 1/2" and 1" osteotome curved 1/2" through 1 1/2" straight osteotomes • straight and gooseneck rongeur • small rongeur • 2 small cup curette • mallet • femoral impactor • tibial impactor • nerve hook • meniscal clamp • 1/2" key elevator • pliers • marking pen	1. Have oscillating saw, power drills, and lavage ready. 2. Check surgeon's preference for implant system.

Triple Arthrodesis of Ankle Setup

Core: Orthopedic	Level II

Clamps	Knives/Scalpels	Scissors	Forceps	Retractors	Miscellaneous	Notes
• 2 curved hemostat • 2 straight Ochsner	• 3 #3 handle with 15 blade	• small Metzenbaum • straight Mayo • single-tooth Adson	• Bonney	• vertebral spreader • Senn • Army–Navy • Hohmann	• 1/4" and 1/2" osteotomes • small rongeur • small curettes • mallet • Freer elevator • 1/4" and 1/2" key elevators • marking pen	1. Have burrs, oscillating saw, power drill, pins, and staples available. 2. Have implant system available.

Ulnar Nerve Transposition Setup

Core: Orthopedic	Level I

Soft-Tissue Hand Procedure setup with the addition of the following instruments.

	Miscellaneous
• 2 small right angles	• high-powered drill and burr • 1/8" Penrose drain, vessel loop, or umbilical tape

Personal Notes

Personal Notes

Personal Notes

Personal Notes

Chapter 9

Neurologic Surgery

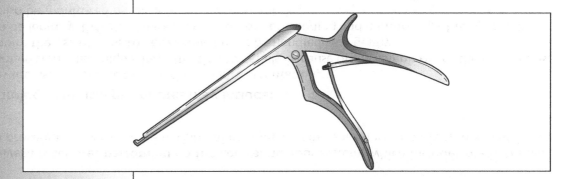

Introduction

Neurologic surgery involves procedures performed on the central nervous system, which includes the brain and the spinal cord, and also procedures involving the peripheral nervous system, which includes the cranial and spinal nerves.

Considerations for neurologic surgical procedures may include:

- This specialty involves the use of specific and specialized instrumentation.
- It is important to maintain sterile technique. Pay attention to details, because of the complexity of the procedures.
- Some procedures require the use of a microscope, which must be handled very gently.
- These procedures can be lengthy, therefore necessitating proper positioning and monitoring of temperature.
- Urinary output may also be monitored because of the use of mannitol.
- Specific sponges (Cottonoids/Patties) are made to be used during neurologic procedures. These are usually moistened with saline and placed in a basin/cup on the Mayo setup for easy access. They may also be moistened with chemical hemostatic agents.
- Because of the delicate tissue involved in these procedures, it is important to protect the tissue with sponges while retracting or suctioning.
- Hemostatic scalp clips may be used during a craniotomy and should be available.
- Special positioning devices, such as head rest, frames, and tables, may be utilized.
- Ultrasonic aspirators may be used for tumor resection.
- A special table called a Mayfield table may be used for Mayo setup because it is larger, can accommodate more supplies, and can be positioned over the patient for easy access.

List of Procedures

Anterior Cervical Discectomy with Fusion Setup

Specialty: Neuro	Level III

Clamps	Knives/Scalpels	Scissors	Forceps	Retractors	Miscellaneous	Notes
• 2 curved hemostat • 2 curved Ochsner with dissectors	• #3 handle with 10 blade • #7 handle with 15 blade	• small Metzenbaum • micro scissors, curved • straight Mayo	• single-tooth Adson • bayonet without teeth • Cushing without teeth • Cushing with teeth	• Weitlaner • Army–Navy	• small pituitary rongeur • Kerrison punch, variety • curettes, small cup, straight and angled • Penfield dissectors, #3 and #4 • Freer elevator • 2 small key elevators • spinal needle • bipolar cautery • marking pen	1. Have burrs or Midas Rex available. 2. If taking a graft from the crest, add gouges, large curettes, osteotomes, mallet, large Weitlaner retractor, and possibly Gelfoam.

Carpal Tunnel Release Setup

Specialty: Neuro	Level I

Clamps	Knives/Scalpels	Scissors	Forceps	Retractors	Miscellaneous
• 2 curved hemostat	• 2 #3 handle with 15 blade	• small Metzenbaum • straight Mayo • tenotomy	• single-tooth Adson	• small Gelpi • small Weitlaner	• marking pen • small bipolar cautery

Craniotomy Setup

Specialty: Neuro	Level III

Clamps	Knives/Scalpels	Scissors	Forceps	Retractors	Miscellaneous	Notes
• 4–6 Dandy • 2 curved hemostat	• #3 handle with 10 blade • #3 handle with 11 blade • #3 handle with 15 blade	• dural • small Metzenbaum • straight suture	• single-tooth Adson • bayonet without teeth • Cushing with teeth	• vein retractor • Cushing • Weitlaner	• Rainey clips and appliers • Penfield dissectors, #1, 2, 3, 4 • 2 Freer elevators with bone wax • small key elevator • small rongeur • small Kerrison punch • dural separator • dural hook • brain spoon • hemostatic clips • marking pen	1. Various sizes of neurologic sponges (Cottonoids) should be moistened with saline and placed in a basin/cup on the Mayo tray. 2. Strips of Gelfoam with thrombin may also be used. 3. Bipolar cautery. 4. Rubber bands. 5. Have drill, burrs, or Midas Rex ready. 6. Setup may also be used for craniectomy and cranioplasty. 7. If being performed for aneurysm clipping, need to have aneurysm clips available. 8. May use microscope.

Lumbar Laminectomy Setup

Specialty: Neuro	Level II

Clamps	Knives/Scalpels	Scissors	Forceps	Retractors	Miscellaneous	Notes
• 2 long straight hemostat • 2 Crile	• #3 handle with 10 blade • #7 handle with 15 blade	• small Metzenbaum • micro • straight Mayo	• single-tooth Adson • bayonet without teeth • Cushing with teeth • Ferris-Smith	• Gelpi • Meyerding • Adson • Weitlaner • nerve root	• pituitary, straight, up and down • small Kerrison punch, straight, angled • Freer elevator with bone wax • blunt nerve hook • 2 Penfield dissectors #4 • 3 Cobb elevator, small, medium, large • curettes, small, medium, large • back-angled curettes, small, medium • rongeur, medium, large • marking pen • a variety of Cottonoids and Gelfoam in thrombin	1. Have available spinal needle, bipolar cautery, Midas Rex. 2. Have a variety of sizes of Cottonoids moistened and in basin on Mayo setup. 3. Strips of Gelfoam with thrombin in a basin.

Transsphenoidal Hypophysectomy Setup

Specialty: Neuro	Level III

Clamps	Knives/Scalpels	Scissors	Forceps	Retractors	Miscellaneous	Notes
• 2 curved hemostat	• sickle • #3 handle with 10 blade • #3 handle with 11 blade • #3 handle with 15 blade	• small Metzenbaum • small straight Mayo • sickle, angled	• DeBakey • Cushing with teeth • bayonet without teeth	• bivalve nasal speculum	• small osteotome • small mallet • sphenoid punch • small ring curette • Hardy's enucleator • pituitary spoon, angled • micro dissectors, angled, straight, curved • Freer elevator • Penfield dissector, #4 • bipolar cautery • hemostatic agents • bone wax • 10 cc syringe with anesthetic of choice	1. May have a separate Mayo setup for graft.

Ventriculoatrial (VA) Shunt or Ventriculoperitoneal (VP) Shunt Setup

Specialty: Neuro	Level II

Clamps	Knives/Scalpels	Scissors	Forceps	Retractors	Miscellaneous	Notes
• 2 curved hemostat • Kelly • vascular	• #3 handle with 10 blade • #3 handle with 11 blade • #3 handle with 15 blade	• dural • small Metzenbaum • Metzenbaum • curved Mayo • straight Mayo	• Cushing • bayonet without teeth • single-tooth Adson	• Richardson • Weitlaner • Army–Navy	• Rainey clips • rubber-shod clamp • tunneling device • 1/4" and 1/2" key elevators • Penfield dissectors, #1, 2, 3 • dural hook • Kerrison punch • bipolar cautery • hemostatic agents • Patties	1. Have shunt system ready.

Personal Notes

Personal Notes

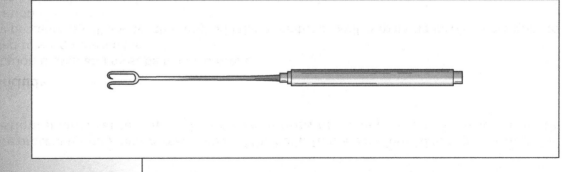

Introduction

Plastic and reconstructive procedures may involve many areas of the body. They are performed to correct congenital anomalies, correct disfigurements caused by pathologic conditions or trauma, and to improve cosmetic appearance.

Considerations may include:

- Delicate instrumentation is used and must be handled properly.
- Scales may be needed to weigh specimens.
- Most plastic surgery procedures will involve the surgeon taking photos as well as marking incision lines prior to beginning the operation.
- These procedures can be lengthy and patients need to be properly padded and protected from exposure.
- Microscopes are often used during plastic surgery procedures; therefore, the Mayo setup may vary to include microscopic instrumentation.
- Grafts and implants may be used.
- When performing skin grafts, it is sometimes important to utilize two Mayo setups or keep the recipient site instrumentation separate from the donor site instrumentation.
- As local anesthetics are often used, syringes and hypodermic needles will be needed.
- Be sure to label all medications on the sterile field.
- As with other specialties, patient confidentiality is of utmost importance.
- Because this specialty includes correction of congenital deformities, it is important to remember that every patient needs support and understanding.
- Surgical dressings for this specialty are designed for various areas of the body in order to reduce risk of infection, as well as to keep the surgical wound clean and covered. Most plastic surgeons have various materials and unique ways in which they dress surgical wounds. This is vital to the postoperative care of flaps and reconstructive procedures.

List of Procedures

Abdominoplasty Setup

Specialty: Plastics	Level II

Clamps	Knives/Scalpels	Scissors	Forceps	Retractors	Miscellaneous
• 4 curved hemostat • 6 straight Ochsner • 2 Kelly • 4 Allis • 2 sponge forceps with 4 × 4 sponges • 2 curved Ochsner with dissectors	• #3 handle with 15 blade • #3 handle with 10 blade	• Metzenbaum • curved and straight Mayo	• Brown multi-tooth • single-tooth	• 2 Army–Navy • 2 small and 2 medium Richardson • 2 blunt prong rake • 1 large Richardson • 1 narrow and 1 medium Deaver	• marking pen • ruler

Augmentation Mammoplasty Repair Setup

Specialty: Plastics	**Level II**

Clamps	Knives/Scalpels	Scissors	Forceps	Retractors	Miscellaneous	Notes
• 2 curved hemostat • 2 straight hemostat • 2 Allis • 2 sponge forceps loaded with 4 × 4 sponges	• 2 #3 handle with 15 blade	• Metzenbaum • tenotomy • straight Mayo	• Brown multi-tooth • Adson single-tooth	• 2 skin hook • 2 double-prong hook	• cautery needle tip and extension • marking pen • ruler • Luer-lock syringe, 27 gauge needle, and surgeon's preference of local anesthetic • areola marker	1. Some surgeons use fiberoptic lighted retractors for this procedure.

Blepharoplasty Setup

Specialty: Plastics	Level I

Clamps	Knives/Scalpels	Scissors	Forceps	Retractors	Miscellaneous
• 4 curved mosquito	• #3 handle with 15 blade • Beaver blade and handle	• Brown dissecting • tenotomy • straight iris	• Brown–Adson • dressing • jeweler	• 2 skin hooks • 2 single-prong and 2 double-prong rake • 2 Blair retractors	• Frazier suction tip • ruler • bipolar cautery forceps • marking pen • local anesthetic and syringe / injection needle • Castroviejo needle holder • Wekcel sponges

Cleft Lip/Palate Repair Setup

Specialty: Oral	Level II

Clamps	Knives/Scalpels	Scissors	Forceps	Retractors	Miscellaneous
• 4 curved mosquito hemostat • 1 Allis • 2 straight hemostat	• #3 handle with 15 blade • #5 Beaver scalpel and blade	• iris • tenotomy • fine-tip Metzenbaum • small straight Mayo	• 2 pair DeBakey • 2 Adson tissue (1 with teeth and 1 smooth)	• 2 skin hook • 2 double-prong hook • palate hook • palate elevators • mouth gag and retractor blades	• Frazier suction tip • lip clamp • caliper • ruler • syringe, local injection needle, and local anesthetic • marking pen • Q-tips® • tongue depressor

Full-Thickness Skin Graft (FTSG) Setup

Specialty: Plastics	Level II

Clamps	Knives/Scalpels	Scissors	Forceps	Miscellaneous	Notes
• 2 curved hemostat • 2 Allis	• #3 handle with 15 blade	• Metzenbaum • suture	• smooth • single-tooth Adson	• dermatome • cord • blade • tongue blade • marking pen • mineral oil	1. Have available mesher and tissue carrier. 2. Mayo setup may also be used for: split-thickness skin graft.

Liposuction Setup

| Specialty: Plastic | Level I |

Knives/Scalpels	Forceps	Miscellaneous	Notes
• 2 #3 handle with 15 blade	• 2 pair Adson tissue with teeth	• suture of surgeon's preference • suction tubing and cannula • needle holder	1. Liposuction procedures are often performed in a doctor's office or as an outpatient procedure.

Reduction Mammoplasty Setup

Specialty: Plastics	Level II

Clamps	Knives/Scalpels	Scissors	Forceps	Retractors	Miscellaneous
• 2 curved hemostat • 2 straight hemostat • 2 Allis	• 2 #3 handle with 15 blade	• Metzenbaum • tenotomy • straight Mayo	• Brown multi-tooth • Adson single-tooth	• 2 skin hook • 2 double-prong hook	• cautery needle tip and extension • marking pen • ruler • Luer-lock syringe, 27 gauge needle, and surgeon's preference of local anesthetic • areola marker

Rhytidectomy Setup

Specialty: Plastics	Level II

Clamps	Knives/Scalpels	Scissors	Forceps	Retractors	Miscellaneous
• 4 curved hemostat • 4 Allis • Burlisher	• 2 #3 handles with 15 blade	• tenotomy • Metzenbaum • suture	• Cushing tissue • 2 pair Brown–Adson	• 2 double-prong hook • 2 single-prong hook • 2 small Deaver • 2 Army–Navy	• syringe, 27 gauge needle, and local anesthetic of surgeon's choice • bipolar cautery • marking pen

Tendon Repair Setup

Specialty: Plastics	Level I

Clamps	Knives/Scalpels	Scissors	Forceps	Retractors	Miscellaneous
• 2 mosquito hemostat • 2 curved hemostat • 2 Allis • 2 right angle	• 2 #3 handle with 15 blade	• short Metzenbaum • small straight Mayo • tenotomy	• DeBakey • Brown multi-tooth • Adson single-tooth	• double-prong hook • 2 Senn • 2 skin hook	• marking pen • Keith needle • needle tip cautery

Personal Notes

Personal Notes

Chapter 11

Ear, Nose, and Throat (ENT or Otorhinolaryngologic) Surgery

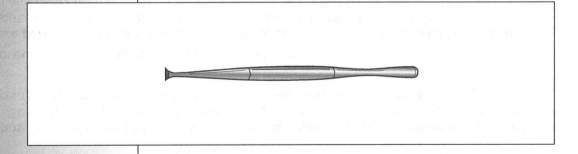

Introduction

ENT surgeries involve those performed on the ear, nose, and throat regions. Surgical intervention may be done to correct congenital abnormalities, repair structural defects caused by trauma or disease, and to restore function of organs. Pharmaceutical agents that are used should be labeled. Monopolar or bipolar cautery devices may be used.

Considerations for procedures performed on the ear may include:

- Most ear surgeries are performed through operating microscopes. The scrub person will be handling delicate microscopic instruments and will have to guide them to the surgeon's hands for use. It is important to keep instruments organized and ready for use.
- The scrub person needs to be able to assemble the various power drills and saws that will be used.
- A wide variety of grafts may be used to replace membranes or ossicles.

Considerations for nasal procedures may include:

- Nasal procedures may be performed using an endoscope or with an open incision.
- On most procedures, a separate Mayo setup is used prior to the operation for injection and topical application of local anesthetics.
- Cottonoid sponges (Neuro patties) are often used, as are different hemostatic agents.

Considerations for procedures performed on the throat may include:

- Surgeons may require special headlights.
- Long or specialized instruments may be needed.
- Special sponges with strings attached are used in the throat region.
- A special suction/cautery device may be used.
- If working with the larynx, a microscope and laser may be used.

Considerations for ENT procedures may include:

- ENT surgery also utilizes special knives/blades such as the Beaver knife and a 12 blade on a #7 handle.
- ENT surgical procedures are commonly performed on children. This necessitates the precautions followed when dealing with children, such as warm rooms, communication, "child friendly" equipment, and so forth.

List of Procedures

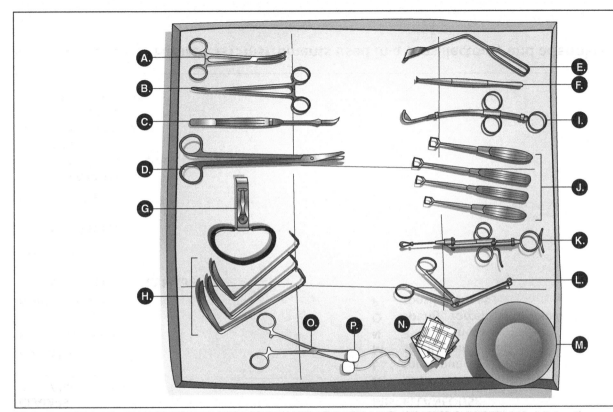

Figure 11-1: Instruments used in a tonsillectomy and adenoidectomy

CLAMPS:

A   Allis

FORCEPS:

B   tonsil forceps

KNIVES/SCALPELS:

C   #7 handle with 12 blade

SCISSORS:

D   tonsil scissors

RETRACTORS:

E   uvula retractor
F   Hurd–Pilar retractor
G   mouth gag
H   tongue depressor
I   adenotome
J   adenoid curette

MISCELLANEOUS:

K   tonsil snare
L   tonsil punch
M   small basin
N   3 × 3 sponges
O   sponge forceps with tonsil sponges
P   tonsil sponges

Key to Accompany Figure 11-1: Instruments used in a tonsillectomy and adenoidectomy

Adenoidectomy Setup

Core: ENT	Level I

Clamps	Scissors	Forceps	Retractors	Miscellaneous
• 1 Kelly • 1 Schnidt tonsil • 2 sponge forceps	• straight Mayo	• Brown multi-tooth	• Davis mouth gag	• mirror • anti-fog • tonsil sponges • Barnhill curettes • Adenoid punch • 16 red rubber catheter

Caldwell–Luc Procedure Setup

Core: ENT	Level II

Knives/Scalpels	Scissors	Forceps	Retractors	Miscellaneous	Notes
• #3 handle with 15 blade	• small Metzenbaum	• Adson–Brown • bayonet	• Caldwell–Luc	• Freer elevator • small osteotome • mallet • small Kerrison rongeur • Coakley curettes • Takahashi pituitary rongeur • antrum trocar/rasp • insulated suction cautery • local anesthetic of surgeon's preference • drill	1. This Mayo setup can be used for internal maxillary artery ligation with the addition of a ligating-hemostatic clip.

Fiberoptic Endoscopic Sinus Surgery (FESS) Setup

Core: ENT	Level I

Knives/Scalpels	Scissors	Forceps	Miscellaneous	
• #3 handle with 15 blade	• nasal • endoscopic	• nasal (straight and upward bent) • straight and angled Blakesley • polyp	• antrum punch • scope sheaths • telescopes: 1, 25, and 70 degree • Coakley antrum curette • suction/irrigator • pharmaceuticals • anti-fog • fluid tubing • camera • light cord	**Second Mayo Tray Setup:** • topical and local anesthetic • Q-tip® applicators • sponges • nasal speculum • bayonet forceps

Frontal Sinus Obliteration Setup

Core: ENT	Level II

Clamps	Knives/Scalpels	Scissors	Forceps	Retractors	Miscellaneous	
• 2 curved hemostat	• 2 #3 handle with 15 blade	• small Metzenbaum • small straight Mayo	• single-tooth Adson • bayonet • DeBakey • straight fine	• Weitlaner	• Freer elevator • periosteal elevator • small curette • small rongeur • small osteotome • Kerrison punch • rasp • small mallet • Raney clips and appliers • saw with oscillating blade • bone wax • marking pen • frontal rasp • blunt nerve hook • dural hook	**Second Mayo Tray Setup:** • topical and local anesthetic • Q-tip® applicators • sponges • nasal speculum • bayonet forceps

Laryngoscopy Setup

Core: ENT	Level I

Knives/Scalpels	Forceps	Miscellaneous	Notes
• laryngeal knives	• biopsy • laryngeal grasping • laryngeal cup • laryngeal alligator	• laryngoscope • laryngeal suction tips • mouth guard • laryngeal mirror • Luken trap • lubricant • hypodermic needle • light cord • scope suction • microscope • laryngoscope holder • tooth guard • medicine cup with warm water	1. If using a microscope, you will need to add: microscopic instrumentation such as scissors, forceps, knives, probe, and microlaryngeal mirror.

Mentoplasty Setup

Core: ENT	Level I

Clamps	Knives/Scalpels	Scissors	Forceps	Retractors	Miscellaneous	Notes
• 4 curved hemostat • 2 straight hemostat • 2 mosquito	• #3 handle with 15 blade	• tenotomy • iris	• 2 pair Adson multi-tooth • DeBakey	• 2 skin hook • 2 Senn	• marking pen • Freer elevator	1. Have various size implants available.

Myringotomy with Pressure Equalization (PE) Tubes Setup

Core: ENT	Level I

Miscellaneous	Notes
• ear specula • ear curettes • ear loop • sexton knife • Frazier suction tip • alligator forceps • PE tube applicator • PE tubes • cotton balls • 3 × 3 sponges	1. Microscope will be used.

Parotidectomy Setup

Core: ENT		Level II	

Clamps	Knives/Scalpels	Scissors	Forceps	Retractors	Miscellaneous
• 4 curved mosquito • 2 curved hemostat • 2 Allis • 2 Kelly • 2 right angle	• #3 handle with 15 blade	• Metzenbaum • tenotomy • straight Mayo	• Adson multi-tooth • Adson single-tooth	• 2 rake • 2 skin hook • 2 Army–Navy	• sterile nerve stimulator • hemoclips

Radical Neck Dissection Setup

Core: ENT	Level III

Clamps	Knives/Scalpels	Scissors	Forceps	Retractors	Miscellaneous	Notes
• 6 small curved hemostat • 4 curved hemostat • 2 small vascular • 2 right angle • 1 Allis • 1 Kelly • 2 curved Ochsner with dissectors	• #7 handle with 15 blade • #3 handle with 10 blade	• Metzenbaum • straight Mayo • sharp dissecting	• bayonet • single-tooth • 2 pair DeBakey • Brown multi-tooth	• Green retractor • 2 skin hook • 2 vein • 2 Weitlaner	• nerve stimulator • vessel loops • marking pen • 10 cc syringe with 25 gauge needle • pharmaceuticals of surgeon's preference	1. Have tracheostomy set and tubes available. 2. Mayo setup may also be used for: parotidectomy.

Submucous Resection Setup

Core: ENT	Level I

Knives/Scalpels	Scissors	Forceps	Retractors	Miscellaneous	Notes
• #3 handle with 15 blade • #7 handle with 15 blade • swivel	• small straight Mayo • Metzenbaum • tenotomy • iris	• bayonet • thumb • dressing • Cottle • Takahashi • nasal cutting • Jansen–Middleton	• 2 skin hook • 2 Joseph hook	• nasal speculum • Freer elevator • chisel • Kerrison rongeur • rasp • Cottonoids • bone crusher on back table **Second Mayo Tray Setup:** • topical and local anesthetic • Q-tip® applicators • sponges • nasal speculum • bayonet forceps	1. Mayo setup may also be used for: rhinoplasty.

Tonsillectomy and Adenoidectomy Setup

Core: ENT	Level I

Clamps	Forceps	Knives/Scalpels	Scissors	Retractors	Miscellaneous
• 2 tonsil Allis	• tonsil • 2 Schnidt tonsil artery	• #7 handle with 12 blade	• tonsil	• uvula • Hurd–Pilar • mouth gag • tongue depressor	• tonsil snare • tonsil punch • small basin • adenotome • adenoid curette • 3 × 3 sponges • sponge forceps with tonsil sponge • insulated cautery/suction device • tonsil sponges

Tympanoplasty Setup

Core: ENT	Level II

Clamps	Knives/Scalpels	Scissors	Forceps	Retractors	Miscellaneous	Notes
• 2 curved mosquito hemostat • 2 straight mosquito hemostat	• #3 handle with 15 blade • House tympanoplasty knife • roller knife • Beaver knife • sickle knife	• small curved • small straight Mayo • Bellucci	• Adson with teeth • bayonet • House Gelfoam • cup	• 2 Senn • mastoid • 2 skin hook • 2 Weitlaner	• ear speculum • mastoid curette • mastoid gouges • malleus nipper • ruler • drum elevator • pick—45 and 90 degree • bone wax • Gelfoam • tongue blade • micro wipe • 5 mL syringe • drill • burrs • suction/irrigations • local anesthetic • 3 mL syringe • 1 mL syringe • pharmaceuticals of surgeon's choice • bipolar forceps • Gelfoam press • duckbill elevator	1. Mayo setup may also be used for: stapedectomy (you will need to add implants).

Uvulopalatopharyngoplasty (UPPP) Setup

Core: ENT	Level I

Clamps	Knives/Scalpels	Scissors	Retractors	Miscellaneous	Notes
• 2 Schnidt tonsil • 2 Allis	• #7 handle with 12 or 15 blade	• Metzenbaum	• Davis mouth gag	• Hurd dissector • Colver tonsil-grasping forceps • ENT suction and cautery • tonsil sponges • mirror • anti-fog • tonsil tenaculum	1. Have headlight available. 2. May be performed with laser (follow safety protocol). 3. Have tracheostomy supplies available. 4. Tonsillectomy may also be performed.

Personal Notes

Personal Notes

Personal Notes

Chapter 12

Ophthalmic Surgery

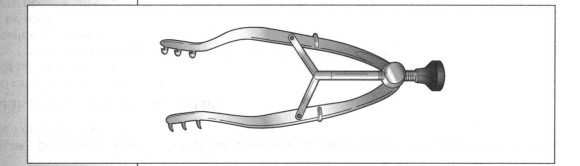

Introduction

Ophthalmic surgery involves procedures done on the globe, orbit, muscles, and the lacrimal system. It is done to restore the patient's vision or for plastic repairs.

Considerations for ophthalmic procedures may include:

- Microscopes are used on almost every procedure.
- Materials used should be lint free.
- Sterile gloves must be rinsed free of glove powder prior to beginning the procedure.
- Sponges are precut cellulose on sticks.
- Bipolar cautery may be used.
- Disposable eye cautery pencil is often used.
- Local anesthetics and solutions will be on the Mayo setup and should be properly labeled.
- Instrumentation is extremely delicate. The scrub person should check sharp edges before surgery and make sure all instruments are in functioning order.
- The scrub person should also have knowledge of drills, burs, and specialized nasal instruments that might be used on procedures involving the lacrimal system.
- Specialized equipment may be used for cataract extractions. They should be functioning properly.
- Do not handle the lens with gloved hands; glove powder can be damaging to the eye.
- Ophthalmic procedures are commonly performed under a local anesthetic, so it is necessary to keep the room quiet for the patient's comfort.

List of Procedures

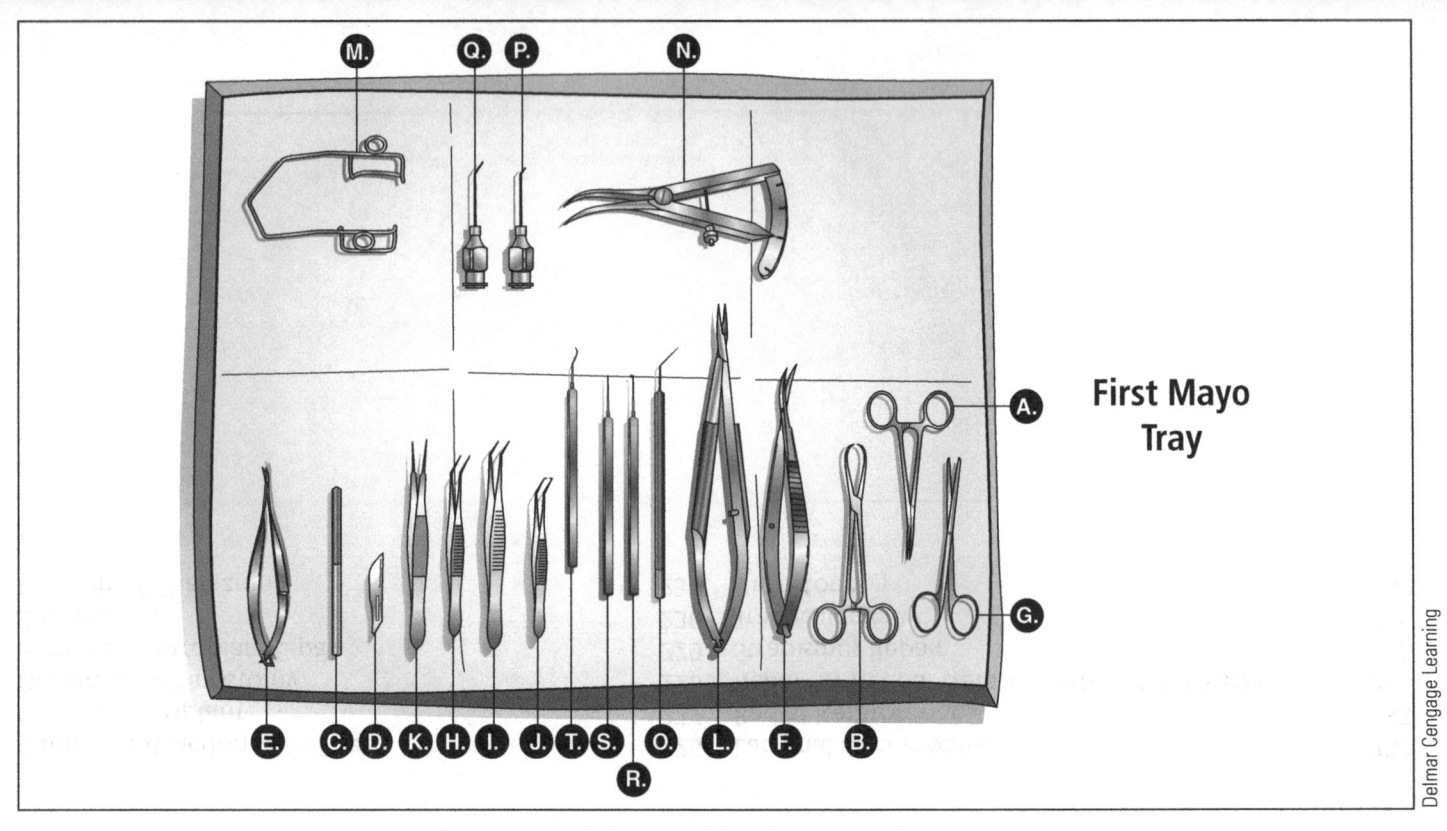

First Mayo Tray

Figure 12-1: Instruments used in a cataract extraction with phaco

CLAMPS:

A   curved hemostat
B   small towel clip

KNIVES/SCALPELS:

C   Beaver knife handles
D   75 Beaver blade

SCISSORS:

E   Vannas curved scissors
F   sharp and dull Westcott scissors
G   straight strabismus suture scissors

FORCEPS:

H   Kelman–McPherson forceps
I   tying forceps
J   superior rectus forceps
K   0.12 forceps

MISCELLANEOUS:

L   titanium needle holder
M   Barraquer eye speculum
N   Castroviejo caliper
O   Bechert nucleus rotator
P   27g air injection cannula
Q   19g irrigation cannula
R   Kuglen iris hook
S   Sinskey lens hook
T   Clayman guide

Key to Accompany Figure 12-1: Instruments used in a cataract extraction with phaco

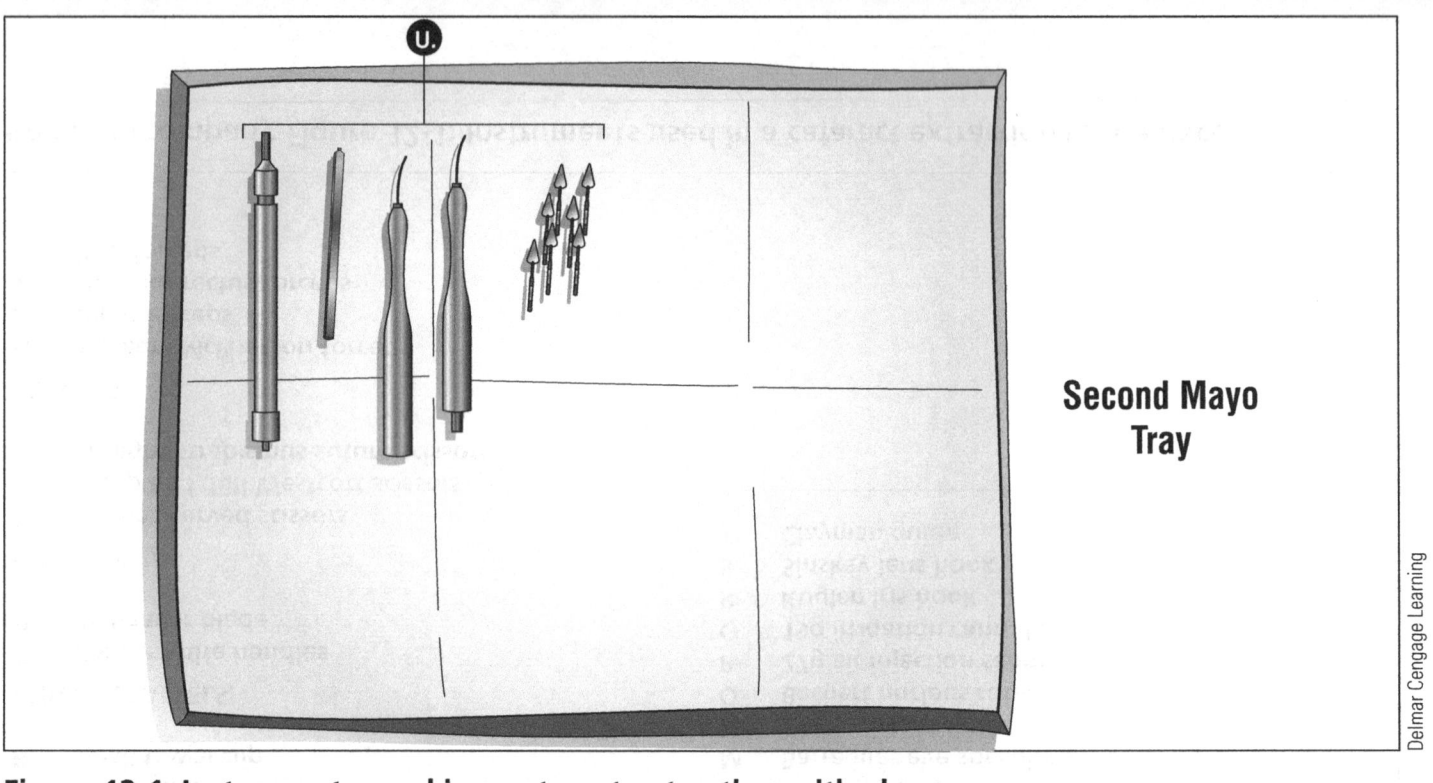

Second Mayo Tray

Figure 12-1: Instruments used in a cataract extraction with phaco

MISCELLANEOUS:

U   Phaco handpiece, cystotome handle, irrigation and aspiration

Key to Accompany Figure 12-1: Instruments used in a cataract extraction with phaco

Cataract Extraction with Phaco Setup

Specialty: Opthalmic	Level II

Clamps	Knives/Scalpels	Scissors	Forceps	Miscellaneous	Notes
• curved hemostat • small towel clip	• Beaver knife handles • 75 Beaver blade • keratome	• Vannas curved • sharp and dull Westcott • straight strabismus suture	• Kelman–McPherson • tying • superior rectus • capsulorhexis • 0.12 forceps	• cyclodialysis spatula • titanium needle holder • Barraquer eye speculum • Castroviejo caliper • Bechert nucleus rotator • 27g air injection cannula • 19g irrigating cannula • Kuglen iris hook • Sinskey lens hook • Clayman guide	1. Have balanced saline solution (BSS) drops, cellulose sponges, and tetrocaine ready. 2. On a second Mayo setup you will need the following: phaco handpiece, cystotome handle, and irrigation and aspiration.

Corneal Transplant Setup

Specialty: Opthalmic	Level II

Two Mayo setups are used for this procedure.

First Mayo setup

Knives/Scalpels	Scissors	Forceps	Miscellaneous		Notes
• 75 Beaver blade on handle	• corneal, left and right • Vannas	• 0.12 forceps • Castroviejo suturing • Bishop–Harmon • Colibri corneal	• Castroviejo needle holders • Barraquer eye speculum • Green strabismus hook • Troutman corneal dissector • universal trephine handle • disposable trephine blades • Flieringa fixation rings (size 12 mm–22 mm) • Paton spatula • BSS with 19g needle • air cannula, 27g	**Second Mayo Tray table setup:** • Cup for cornea • 0.12 forceps • BSS • corneal button punch • corneal block • extra gloves	1. Have cellulose sponges, antibiotics, and eye pad available.

Dacryocystorhinostomy Setup

Specialty: Opthalmic	Level II

Clamps	Knives/Scalpels	Scissors	Forceps	Retractors	Miscellaneous	Notes
• 2 mosquito hemostat	• #3 handle with 15 blade • #3 handle with 11 blade	• straight and curved tenotomy	• 0.5 forceps • 0.3 forceps • bayonet • Castroviejo suturing	• 2 Senn rake • lid sac	• nose speculum • Freer elevators • Muldoon elevator • Worst pigtail probe • small rongeur • lacrimal probes and dilators • small Kerrison punch • lacrimal gouges • lacrimal osteotomes • small mallet • lacrimal duct intubation set • lid clamp • bipolar forceps	1. Have power drills and burrs ready, as well as bone wax. 2. Separate Mayo setup will be used for nasal preparation.

Ectropian/Entropian Repair Setup

Specialty: Opthalmic	Level I

Clamps	Knives/Scalpels	Scissors	Forceps	Retractors	Miscellaneous	Notes
• 4 mosquito hemostat • Serrentine	• #3 handle with 15 blade • #9 handle with 11 blade	• Castroviejo corneal • curved and straight iris • intraocular vitrectomy • Stevens • Wescott	• Castroviejo suturing • fixation • 1 straight and 1 curved extra fine serrated	• eye speculum • Green muscle hooks • iris hook	• Barraquer needle holder • Troutman-Barraquer needle holder • marking pen • cotton tip applicators • eye pad and shield • iris spatula • wet bipolar	1. Fiber optic microscope is often used. 2. Basic eye microscope tray is needed. 3. Eyelid procedure tray should be available.

Enucleation Setup

Specialty: Opthalmic	Level I

Clamps	Scissors/Scalpels	Forceps	Retractors	Miscellaneous
• small curved hemostat	• curved enucleation	• 0.3 forceps • 0.5 forceps • recession	• Arruga orbital • lacrimal sac	• Lancaster eye speculum • enucleation spoon • small Kerrison punch • Freer elevator • exenteration spoon • serrefine • muscle hooks • enucleation snare • sphere prosthesis and conformers • sphere introducer and holder • BSS, cellulose sponges, and antibiotics

Excision of Chalazion Setup

Knives/Scalpels	Forceps	Miscellaneous
• #3 handle with 11 blade	• 0.12 forceps	• Desmarres chalazion clamp • chalazion curettes • short Q-tips® • plain sponges • BSS

Lacrimal Duct Probing Setup

Specialty: Opthalmic	Level I

Forceps	Miscellaneous
• 0.12 forceps	• lacrimal probe and dilators • 3 × 3 sponges • 2–3 cc syringes • irrigation tips • 27 gauge air needles • fluorescein dye • lacrimal cannulas • Freer elevator • safety pin

Radial Keratotomy Setup

Knives/Scalpels	Forceps	Miscellaneous
• sapphire knife • diamond knife	• corneal fixation • Castroviejo–Colibri 0.12 • Bores incision-spreading	• fixation device • Barraquer speculum • Bores corneal knife gauge • depth gauge • corneal marker • elliptical optic center marker • Castroviejo caliper • air cannula, 27 gauge • BSS, cellulose sponges, and antibiotics

Repair of Retinal Detachment—Scleral Buckling Setup

Specialty: Opthalmic	Level II

Knives/Scalpels	Scissors	Forceps	Retractors	Miscellaneous
• 59 or 69 Beaver blade	• Westcott blunt • tenotomy • utility • Stevens straight	• 0.5 forceps • angled Nugent • tying • Bonaccolto • Bishop with teeth	• Schepens • lid	• cryoprobe • Castroviejo needle holder • Castroviejo caliper • Gonian marker • Schiotz tonometer • muscle hook • silicone implant • BSS and antibiotics, cellulose sponges

Strabismus Repair Setup

Specialty: Opthalmic	Level I

Clamps	Knives/Scalpels	Scissors	Forceps	Retractors	Miscellaneous
• small curved hemostat	• #9 handle with 15 or 11 blade	• sharp and dull Westcott • straight and curved Strabismus	• 0.3 forceps • 0.5 forceps • fixation • recession • bipolar	• lacrimal sac • eye speculum	• Castroviejo caliper • serrefine • Jameson muscle hook, small and large • caliper • needle holder • BSS with 19 gauge needle, cotton-tipped applicators, cellulose sponges, and antibiotics

Trabeculectomy Setup

Specialty: Opthalmic	Level II

Clamps	Knives/Scalpels	Scissors	Forceps	Retractors	Miscellaneous	Notes
• 4 mosquito hemostat • 2 Serrefine	• #57 Beaver blade • 15 degree super blade	• Wescott • Stevens • iris	• small smooth • diathermy • bipolar wet field diathermy • corneal • Bonn	• eyelid speculum • iris hook	• Castroviejo needle holder • 4-0 or 5-0 traction suture • Von Graefe hook • basic eye procedure tray • glaucoma procedures tray • marking pen • iris spatula • eye pad and shield • antibiotic drops	1. Iridectomy may also be performed.

Vitrectomy Setup

Specialty: Opthalmic | **Level III**

	Forceps	Miscellaneous
Cataract extraction setup with the following additions: • Vannas scissors • Nylon suture • Vitreous	• Lister • Pierse–Hoskins, curved and straight • McPherson tying • foreign body • scleral plug	• vitrectomy handpiece and tubing • scleral plugs (19 or 20g) • handheld lens (with irrigator) • caliper • infusion cannula • membrane pick • flute needle • BSS, sodium hyaluronate, vitreous substitute, cotton-tipped applicators, acetylcholine, antibiotics, and cellulose sponges

Personal Notes

Personal Notes

Personal Notes

Chapter 13

Oral/ Maxillofacial Surgery

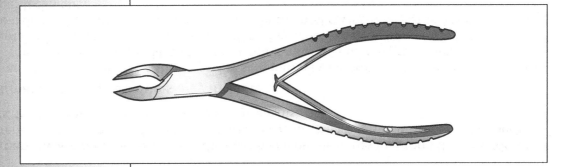

Introduction

Oral and maxillofacial surgery involve procedures done in the mouth and on the bones that form the face. Most surgeries are performed to repair fractures and deformities, and to remove or replace teeth. Instrumentation includes typical dental instruments, fracture sets, and orthopedic-style instruments.

Considerations for oral/maxillofacial procedures may include:

- When dealing with craniofacial deformities, other specialty surgeons may be involved such as neuro, plastic or ophthalmic surgeons. You would add the specialized instrumentation for that region/procedure.
- Dental drills, burs, dental rolls, anti-fog, dental mirrors, and local injections may be used. Although this instrumentation will not remain sterile once the procedure begins on the oral cavity, it is best to keep it surgically clean and follow proper technique.
- For restoration procedures, the scrub person should know how to work with amalgam or resin.
- During maxillofacial procedures, the scrub person should have implants ready, such as plates, screws, or wire according to surgeon's preference. You may also need to use grafts for bone loss. These grafts may be from the patient, so instrumentation for graft harvest may be required. Antibiotic solution should be available.
- This specialty may include temporomandibular joint procedures. Consideration here includes knowledge of scopes, cameras, and shaving systems. The video tower system must be checked prior to use.
- Oral surgeons often bring their own technicians to the OR to assist in their procedures.

List of Procedures

Application of Arch Bars Setup

Specialty: Oral/Maxillofacial	Level I

Clamps	Knives/Scalpels	Scissors	Forceps	Retractors	Miscellaneous	Notes
• 2 curved hemostat	• #3 handle with 15 blade	• Dean	• bayonet without teeth • Adson with teeth	• Wieder tongue (large and small) • Minnesota cheek	• Woodson condenser • Freer elevator • V-shaped probe • 2 aspirating syringes • 2 self-cleaning suction tips • wire twister • short and long wire cutter • 2–10 cc syringes with 25g (1/2" needle for local anesthetic) • 2–20 cc syringes with 19g (1" blunt needle for irrigation) • throat pack • gauze sponges • stainless steel wire (24g and 26g) • arch bars • bite block	1. A wire cutter should be sent home with the patient.

Dental Restoration Setup

Specialty: Oral/Maxillofacial | **Level I**

Miscellaneous	Notes
• dental mirror • explorer • cotton plier • burnisher • condenser • amalgam carrier • various burs • high-speed handpiece • slow-speed handpiece • bite block • floss • scaler • flat instrument • amalgam well • amalgam capsules • carver • spoon • carrier • articulating paper	1. May need local anesthetic, syringes, and injection needles. 2. Surgeons may brings their own technicians. 3. Most dental restorations are performed on pediatric patients.

Extraction Setup

Specialty: Oral/Maxillofacial	Level I

Knives/Scalpels	Scissors	Forceps	Retractors	Miscellaneous	Notes
• 2 #3 handle with 15 blade	• Dean • Mayo	• Asch • upper anterior • bayonet • 150, 152 forceps • Cowhorn • smooth	• Pritchard • Minnesota • Wieder	• Woodson condenser • 301, 345, B elevators • tiny basin with peridex • bite block • gauze sponges • dental rolls • throat pack • file • rongeur • osteotome • mallet • Lucas curette • needle holder • 2 self-cleaning tips • dental mirror • local anesthetic with epinephrine • 2–10 cc syringes with 25 gauge 1 1/2" needles • 2–20 cc syringes with 19 gauge 1-1/2" blunt needles	1. Have dental drill ready.

Le Fort I Fracture Repair Setup

Specialty: Oral/Maxillofacial	Level II

Clamps	Knives/Scalpels	Retractors	Miscellaneous	Notes
• 2 curved hemostat	• 2 #7 handle with 15 blade	• Blair	• marking pen • gauze sponges • 2–10 cc syringes with 25 gauge 1-1/2" needles for local anesthetic • 2–20 cc syringes with 19 gauge 1-1/2" blunt needles for irrigation • Freer elevator • periosteal elevator • drill guide • depth guage • wires • wire twister • wire cutter • curette	1. Have arch bars and wires and drill ready. 2. A pair of wire cutters should to be sent home with the patient.

Orbital Floor Fracture Setup

Specialty: Oral/Maxillofacial	Level II

Clamps	Knives/Scalpels	Scissors	Forceps	Retractors	Miscellaneous	Notes
• 2 curved hemostat	• 2 #3 handle with 15 blade	• tenotomy • small Metzenbaum • straight Mayo	• Adson with teeth • bayonet	• Senn • vein	• marking pen • cellulose sponges • 4 × 4 sponges • 2–10 cc syringes with 25 gauge 1-1/2" needle for local anesthetic • 2–20 cc syringes with 19 gauge 1-1/2" blunt needles for irrigation • Freer elevator • periosteal elevator • orbital retractor • curette	1. Have power drill and Silastic sheeting ready. 2. Have rigid fixation set ready—if needed you would add drill guide and depth gauge.

Repair of Mandibular Fracture Setup

Specialty: Oral/Maxillofacial	Level II

Knives/Scissors	Scissors	Forceps	Retractors	Miscellaneous	Notes
• #3 handle with 15 blade • #7 handle with 15 blade	• tenotomy • small Metzenbaum • straight Mayo	• holding • mandibular reduction	• Senn • Joseph skin hook	• throat pack • gauze sponges • 2–10 cc syringes with 25 gauge 1-1/2" needles for local injection • 2–20 cc syringes with 19 gauge 1-1/2" blunt needles for irrigation • small ribbon retractors • Freer elevator • Dingman elevator • Langenbeck elevator • plate holding clamp • drill guide • depth gauge • chisel • mallet • curette • Yankauer suction tip • Frazier tip	1. May need arch bars and wire.

Temporomandibular Joint (TMJ) Arthroscopy Setup

Specialty: Oral/Maxillofacial | **Level I**

Knives	Scissors	Forceps	Miscellaneous	Notes
• #7 handle with 11 blade	• Metzenbaum • tenotomy • straight Mayo	• Adson–Brown	• 30" extension tubing • stopcock • 10 cc and 20 cc syringes • 18 gauge 1-1/2" needle • trocar • cannula • probe • grasper • 0, 30, and 70 degree lens • camera • light cord • shaving system	1. Have ready video tower, shaving system unit, fluid infusion with lactated Ringer's solution.

Personal Notes

Personal Notes

References

A.S.T., Inc. (2001), *Surgical technology for the surgical technologist: A positive care approach,* (1st ed.), Albany, NY: Delmar-Thomson Learning.

Fortunato, N. H. (2000), *Berry & Kohn's operating room technique,* (9th ed.), St. Louis, MO: Mosby.

Goldman, M. (1996), *Pocket guide to the operating room,* (2nd ed.), Philadelphia, PA: F.A. Davis.

Meeker, M.H. and Rothrock, J. (1999), *Alexander's care of the patient in surgery,* (11th ed.), St. Louis, MO: Mosby.

Tighe, S.B. (1999), *Instrumentation for the operating room: A photographic manual,* (5th ed.), St. Louis, MO: Mosby.

Index

Note: Page numbers set in *italic* refer to illustrations.